the art
of Hiding
Vegetables

the art of Hiding Vegetables

sneaky ways to feed your children healthy food

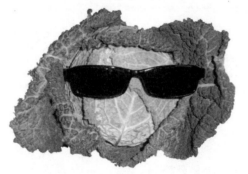

Karen Bali & Sally Child

Editors Richard Craze, Roni Jay

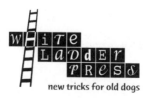

new tricks for old dogs

Published by White Ladder Press Ltd
Great Ambrook, Near Ipplepen, Devon TQ12 5UL
01803 813343
www.whiteladderpress.com

First published in Great Britain in 2005

10 9 8 7 6 5 4 3 2 1

The right of Karen Bali and Sally Child to be identified as authors of this work has been asserted by them in accordance with the Copyright, Designs and Patents Act 1988.

ISBN 0 9548219 2 0

British Library Cataloguing in Publication Data
A CIP record for this book can be obtained from the British Library.

Designed and typeset by Julie Martin Ltd
Cover design by Julie Martin Ltd
Cover photograph by Judy Hedger
Illustrations by Chris Mutter
Printed and bound by TJ International Ltd, Padstow, Cornwall

White Ladder Press
Great Ambrook, Near Ipplepen, Devon TQ12 5UL
01803 813343
www.whiteladderpress.com

With thanks to my wonderful husband for his unfailing support and to my gorgeous, long-suffering children for coping with my erratic hours and kitchen experiments.

Karen Bali

To all my young clients who inspire me and teach me so much.

Sally Child

Acknowledgements

With many thanks to the parents who read through the manuscript for us to make sure we hadn't missed a trick, especially Ginny Cunliffe and Holly Keeling.

Disclaimer

Although this book contains science based information from Sally Child, she would like to clarify that some information and suggestions in this book are a step in the right direction and should not be considered an optimum diet. It is a compromise between an ideal diet and the demands of real life in a busy household.

If your child has any health conditions or you are concerned in any way you should seek advice from your doctor and consider seeing a children's nutritional therapist for individual dietary assessment and advice.

magic breakfast
fuel for learning

Breakfast is vital. After a long night of rest, the fast needs to be broken with good food – preferably slow burning carbohydrate such as porridge or wholemeal toast. Breakfast lifts blood sugar levels and kick-starts the body's metabolism and coaxes the old grey matter into life. Without it, the body simply runs out of energy.

Now, as you would imagine, this is particularly important for young children, seeking to make the most of their time in the classroom. But, shockingly, many school children arrive without breakfast. The Child Poverty Action Group states that for 1 in 4 children, the only hot food they receive is at school. In some schools teachers regularly bring in food from their own pocket, for those children arriving too hungry to learn.

One campaigning charity has been working since 2001 to make a difference in this area. Magic Breakfast delivers free breakfast food to schools in most need. During 2004 the project delivered 70,000 breakfast items, including bagels and breakfast cereals.

There is no charge for the services and there is no 'catch'. The charity has a simple goal – to ensure that every child starts the school day with the right fuel for learning – a nutritious breakfast.

To find out more about Magic Breakfast and how you can help please visit: **www.magicbreakfast.com**.

22 Henrietta Street, LONDON WC2E 8PW
t: 020 7836 5434
e: info@magicbreakfast.com
w: ww.magicbreakfast.com
Registered Charity Number 1102510

Contents

Introduction

A balanced diet with at least five portions of fruit or vegetables every day – we all know the theory and it sounds so easy but putting it into practice is another story…

Many of us struggle to get one or two portions into our fussy little darlings; this is, after all, the 'fast food generation'. The closest some kids get to greens is the football field and they wouldn't know a cabbage if it passed them on a bicycle.

There can hardly be a parent in the western world who hasn't at least once (if not once a day) felt guilty about their child's diet. Working parents without time to cook are especially guilt prone. We may feel that every other parent in the world is carefully selecting organic veg, preparing home cooked meals and serving them to their healthy, fresh faced children, who clean their plates, say thank you and offer to clear the table. Maybe families like this do exist but this book is for real parents of real children living on planet earth in the 21st century – the hard working average parents with a freezer full of fish fingers, a cupboard full of crisps and four week old broccoli wilting in the fridge.

This book is not about having super healthy kids who eat tofu and sprouts every day; it is a realistic guide for busy parents of normal children – a step in the right direction towards healthier eating. Neither is this book intended to scare, lecture or bully parents into guilt and unnecessary hard work – most of us feel guilty enough and work hard enough anyway.

Guilt isn't hard to understand when articles about the state of child health appear in our press almost daily, usually with dramatic headlines such as:

- One in five UK kids overweight
- The return of rickets: Vitamin deficiency disease figures up
- Additives cause behavioural problems in our young
- Diabetes: Kids are getting it too
- Packed lunches fail the nutrition test
- Is low fibre a problem for your child?
- One toddler in eight has anaemia
- Parents may outlive unhealthy kids
- Meet the children who NEVER eat vegetables

Whilst articles like this do scare many parents, and of course make them feel guilty, what is often missing is practical advice on how to improve the situation. In addition to ideas and advice about how to increase the amount of fruit and vegetables in your children's diet, you will also find in here some common sense information about healthy eating in general.

It isn't easy being a parent today with convenience food, kiddies' menus, a multitude of sweets and snacks, takeaways and soft drinks wherever you go. Almost every child wants to have the same as their friends and to eat things that look and taste familiar.

However, just a few little changes to shopping and cooking will bring about significant changes to the health of your children in the long run. We are not talking about a radical overhaul of your family diet in the 'makeover/change your life' mould, just a little easy tweaking that can be introduced as gradually as you like. The best news of all is that your children will hardly notice the subtle changes that will increase their intake of nutritious fruit and vegetables. You are even allowed to leave the advice in this book that you don't have time for or don't think your children will take on board – no one is going to check and you won't lose points. If you manage to make just one or two small changes it's a start, so give yourself a pat on the back. Remember that we are with you every step of the way.

Part 1

Healthier eating
for busy families

Understanding the basic principles and learning just a few tricks and techniques can set your family on its way to a healthier diet.

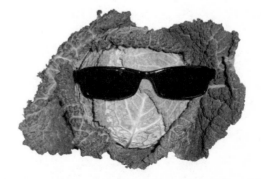

What is healthy eating?

Healthy eating defined

Eating a balanced diet is something we are all encouraged to do, and we often hear that our children also need a balanced diet for health and well-being in the short and long term. Although it's not easy in the 21st century to give children adequate nutrition, by doing so we can give them a good start in life and increase their chances of reaching old age in good health.

But what is a balanced diet and how can parents help children to achieve this? A healthy diet should include some of each of the main food groups, and be varied to provide a wide range of nutrients. As far as is possible, some of this should be 'wholefoods' – basic foods that have not been processed, preserved or refined. Many children consume levels of sugar and salt in their food that are far too high and these should ideally be reduced to within at least the government guidelines (see appendix). Above all, a healthy diet should be interesting, varied, attractive and fun.

The food groups and what they do

Although this book is mostly about fruit and vegetables, their benefits and how to increase intake, they must of course form part of a diet that includes other essential nutrients. These are:

Protein

Much of the protein that children consume usually comes from animal sources, some of which are also high in saturated fat. Sources of protein include meat, fish, soya products, dairy products, eggs, beans and pulses, wholegrains, nuts and quorn. The functions of protein include growth and repair, enzyme and hormone production and energy. Some protein should be consumed with every meal. Many children have low intakes of protein for various reasons; they may find meat difficult to chew, refuse to eat wholegrains or become vegetarian (this quite often happens with teenagers but they do not then replace animal proteins with other sources). Canned fish is a good source of protein, and pulses (including baked beans) also contain protein.

Fats

Children need fats for energy and growth but the word 'fat' sounds negative and things that are low fat are often promoted as healthier. Low fat diets are *not* suitable for children. There are different types of fats and some are 'bad', such as trans-fats or hydrogenated fats. Good sources of fat for children include butter, full fat milk (children under five should always have this rather than skimmed or semi-skimmed milk), lean meat, olive oil, avocados and fish. This food group includes *essential fatty acids* – 'good fats' including the omegas that are mostly found in foods that children often don't eat: nuts, seeds, leafy green vegetables and oily fish. Deficiency in essential fatty acids can lead to learning difficulties, skin problems, constipation, hormone imbalances and weight gain. Omega supplements are often promoted as a way to improve brain function in children. One way to increase natural consumption of essential fatty acids is to finely grind a mixture of nuts and seeds in a blender or coffee grinder and keep the powder in your fridge for a few days to sprinkle on cereal. Alternatively, add oils that contain essential fatty acids – avocado, evening primrose or walnut oils – to cooked rice, pasta, salads or vegetables.

Carbohydrates

There are two types of carbohydrates – simple and complex. Simple carbohydrates are generally found in processed, refined foods such as white bread – sugar is the simplest carbohydrate. Complex carbohydrates come from food containing wholegrains. These contain fibre, protein, minerals and vitamins and are found in foods such as unrefined breakfast cereals, wholemeal bread, oats, brown rice and wholewheat pasta. These carbohydrates are thought to reduce the risk of heart disease, diabetes and digestive cancers. The current fashionable low carb diets should not be considered for children – almost 50% of their diet should consist of carbohydrates, that is, 3-5 servings daily.

Fibre

This is found in fruit and vegetables and also many foods in the carbohydrate group – it is essential for good digestion. However, younger children require lower levels of fibre than adults as their digestion is still developing. High fibre intake in children can reduce the absorption of vitamins and minerals. Fibre is needed for good digestion but as young children cannot metabolise high fibre diets it is best to offer soluble fibre from fruit, veg, salads and wholegrains rather than from too much wheat, for example.

Water

Also essential for health and growth is water. The amount of water children need to consume depends on their age, weight, activity levels and the temperature – more water is required to keep children hydrated in hot weather or warm, stuffy buildings. A one year old child needs around one litre of fluid a day and older children need at least two litres. Adequate water intake is required for brain function, body function and digestion. You can give water in the form of diluted fruit juice. Squash is high in sugar, and the low sugar varieties contain artificial sweeteners which are also a health risk, so it's best to avoid these.

Fruit and vegetables are the last essential food group and this will be described in more detail later in the chapter.

Although an increase in fruit and vegetables and lower levels of sugar consumption are a good thing, it is important to remember that the overall aim is for your children to have a balanced diet. No one food or group of foods can contain everything that children need – they could not thrive on just fruit and vegetables for example. A variety of foods from the different groups provides the nutrients that children need to grow and be healthy.

A word about allergies

Although the information in this book is appropriate for most children, an increasing number of children are born with an allergy or develop intolerance to certain foods for a number of reasons:

- Low vitamin and mineral intake, impaired immune systems due to pollution and toxic overload, consumption of highly processed foods or the limited variety of foods consumed in early childhood.

- Antibiotics and vaccinations may also have an adverse effect on a child's immune system.

- Parents on the whole tend to be more particular about cleaning and 'killing germs' than in previous generations. Play tends to be more sanitised and controlled than it used to be, when making mud pies and catching worms were favourite pastimes for many youngsters. A certain level of dirt and germs, however, can help build immunity.

- Many children also lack 'friendly bacteria' in the digestive tract that can help to prevent allergies and boost immunity.

Allergies tend to be more severe and usually last for life whereas intolerance is acquired due to environmental influences or a compromised immunity. Different antibodies are involved and children may grow out of a food intolerance.

Research into children with allergies has suggested that they are at greater risk of deficiency in vitamins and minerals as their diet may be severely restricted. The most common allergies in children are – wheat, eggs, dairy products, nuts and citrus fruit. If your child suffers from an allergy or intolerance to any of these foods, you will obviously need to modify the advice given in this book. A child who is sensitive to citrus fruit, for example, should not be given this type of fruit in any form, including juice, and other sources of vitamin C should be found instead. If your child has a health problem that is ongoing but has no obvious cause, allergy or intolerance to a particular food may be the cause. Common symptoms of food intolerance are:

- Insomnia
- Learning difficulties
- Unexplained tiredness
- Hyperactivity
- Eczema
- Skin rashes
- Coughs
- Asthma
- Behavioural difficulties
- Low immunity resulting in recurrent infections with slow recovery
- Sore throats
- Headaches
- Tummy ache
- Wind
- Diarrhoea
- Slow growth
- Nausea
- Constipation

A qualified nutritionist will be able to investigate and advise if an allergy or food intolerance is suspected. You might wish to consult your GP or health visitor first – the NHS might test for allergies but they will not test for intolerances.

The benefits of fruit and vegetables

Fruit and vegetables are natural wholefoods that are beneficial in a number of ways:

- They contain *fibre*, both soluble and insoluble, which helps to regulate blood sugar and is good for the digestive system.

- An adequate intake of fruit and vegetables can help to prevent obesity as not only are they mostly high in nutrients and low in calories but will also help children to feel full for longer.

- Fruit and vegetables also have a wide variety of *vitamins* and *minerals*, including those with *anti-oxidant* qualities. This means that in addition to providing the body with vital nutrients, they can reduce cell damage, aid detoxification and boost immunity. Fruits with the highest anti-oxidant qualities are berries (strawberry, blackberry, raspberry) plus dried fruit such as raisins, prunes and apricots. Vegetables high in anti-oxidants include the leafy green varieties (spinach, broccoli, sprouts) and also beetroot and carrots. Tomato products such as purée and ketchup also contain beneficial anti-oxidants in higher levels than raw tomatoes.

Fruit and vegetables contain something unique called *phyto-nutrients*. These are natural plant chemicals that cannot be replicated in any supplement or artificial substance. Phyto-nutrients also come from soya, nuts and pulses but are mainly found in fruit and vegetables. Different types of fruit and vegetables contain different phyto-nutrients, which is why it is important for children to consume a wide variety of colours and types to gain the most benefit. Try to think in terms of colours when deciding on your weekly menu and if possible buy a different selection of fruit and vegetables rather than the same ones each week. The *Rainbow Food Activity Chart* can help children to achieve the right level and variety of fruit and vegetables. It is a colourful wall chart that comes with reusable stickers to help children identify the different colour groups of fruit and vegetables (you'll find details on our website, **www.whiteladderpress.com**, alongside the information about this book).

What is a portion?

What counts as a portion will depend on the age or size of your child – small children obviously require smaller portions of fruit and vegetables than adults. As a general rule, the fruit or vegetable content should account for around 25%-30% of a main meal. A portion for teenagers and adults is roughly 80 grams (approx 3 ounces). There are some foods that many think of as vegetables but should not actually count towards the five a day:

- Potatoes, for example, although they do contain some fibre and vitamins, are mostly starch and do not count as a vegetable.

- Some things count as a portion at a push, but only once a day. For example, fruit juice does count as one, but it lacks fibre and is high in natural sugars so two cups of fruit juice still only counts as one portion.

- Similarly, beans and pulses only count once a day, so five portions of baked beans does not equal five portions (unfortunately).

A variety that includes both fruit and vegetables, raw, cooked, frozen or fresh, of all colours and types (root vegetables, leafy greens, berries, stone fruits etc) makes up the best combination. Tinned fruit and vegetables also count but try to limit to a maximum of one portion a day as they have been heat treated during processing, which can result in loss of nutrients. Wash or peel non-organic fruit and vegetables before cooking or eating to remove any pesticides – the best way to do this is to put 1 table-spoon of vinegar in a bowl of warm water then immerse, and rub dry. Boiling vegetables in water for too long can result in losing most of the nutrients so steam, microwave, stir-fry or cook them for a short time in a little water.

Although five portions a day is the recommended amount of fruit and vegetables, this is the minimum so it is perfectly acceptable to give more if you can manage it. Also, the intake does not neces-sarily need to consist of five individual portions of the same size. Portions can also be smaller in quantity but larger in number. Ten half-portions, for example, may be easier to get down over the course of a day than five whole ones. However, any increase, even from one portion to two, is a step in the right direction. Equally, one large helping of a favourite food can be more than a single portion (although if you do this too often it can be hard to give your child enough variety).

The suggestions on the following pages for portions that count in different age groups may help you to choose.

Supplements

Vitamin and mineral supplements cannot compensate for a poor diet and do not replicate all the qualities of good food. They are designed to *supplement* a good diet to ensure an intake of vital nutrients, not to replace fruit and vegetables as part of a balanced diet. Certain beneficial aspects of foods can be replicated but phyto-nutrients cannot. So why are supplements sometimes necessary?

• Much of the food we eat today is processed, meaning that many of the benefits of wholefoods are lost.

- Intensive farming can mean that soil our food grows in has been depleted of beneficial qualities that should be present in the plants it produces.

- It is very difficult to maintain a balanced diet when parents are busy, if children are fussy eaters or have an erratic appetite.

- Even 'fresh' food may be days or even weeks old by the time we purchase and prepare it – often it is harvested unripe then transported, stored and sold much later. Nutrients are lost without the natural ripening process.

- Pollution is higher than ever in some areas and young bodies need optimum immune systems to cope with fighting it.

- At times of extra growth and development the body uses up its stores of nutrients more rapidly than they can be taken in.

- Some substances cannot be stored in the body so they need to be replaced regularly.

- Research has shown that children who take supplements regularly (in addition to eating fruit and vegetables and avoiding processed food and additives) improve in behaviour becoming less moody and aggressive.

- An optimum level of nutrients may help learning ability.

Supplements should ideally be taken regularly and with food so that they can work together. Both vitamins and minerals are equally important for long term health and well-being.

In addition to vitamins and minerals, supplements of *essential fatty acids* such as omegas 3, 6 and 9 will help keep children healthy.

One supplement that goes some way to imitating the natural benefits of fruit and vegetables is called Kidgreenz by Nature's Plus and is available by mail order or online via the Nutri Centre (see the 'useful contacts' list on our website, **www.whiteladder press.com**, alongside the information about this book).

	1-4 years	5-7 years	8-11 years	12-adult years
Portion Sizes				
baby beetroot	N/A	2	3	4
baby sweetcorn cobs	3	4	4	5-6
banana	1/2 small	1/2 small	1 small	1 large
broccoli/cauliflower	1 floret	2 florets	3 florets	4 florets
celery	N/A	1/2 stick	1 stick	1-2 sticks
grapefruit	N/A	1/2	1/2	1/2
cherry tomatoes	2	3	4	5 or lge
coleslaw	1 tbsp	2 tbsp	3 tbsp	3-4 tbsp
cooked leafy green vegetables	1/2-1 tbsp	1-2tbsp	2-3tbsp	3 tbsp
cooked pulses	1/4 cup	1/2 cup	3/4 cup	1 cup
cooked sliced carrots	1/2 tbsp	1 tbsp	2 tbsp	3 tbsp
cooked vegetables eg beans, etc	1-2 tbsp	2 tbsp	2-3 tbsp	3-4 tbsp
cucumber	2-3 slices	3-4 slices	4-6 slices	6 slices
dried apricots	3	4	6	6-8
fruit juice	50ml	50ml	75ml	100ml
grapes	8	10	12	15
grated carrot	1 tbsp	1 tbsp	2 tbsp	3 tbsp
kiwi fruit	1	2	2	2

	1-4 years	5-7 years	8-11 years	12-adult years
	Portion Sizes			
large fruits eg orange, apple, pear	1/2	1 med	1 med –1 lge	1 lge
melon	25gm slice	50gms	50gms	100gms
mixed fresh fruit salad	1/2 dessert dish	1 dessert dish	1 dessert dish	1 lge dessert
mixed salad	1/2 sm dish	sm dish	1/2 cereal bowl	1 cereal bowl
peach	1/2	1	1	1
peas	1 tbsp	2 tbsp	2 tbsp	3 tbsp
plum	1	1	2	2-3
raisins	1 tbsp	2 tbsp	2 tbsp	handful
raspberries, blackberries, blackcurrants	1-2 tbsp	2 tbsp	3 tbsp	4 tbsp
satsuma	1	1	1-2	2
sliced mushrooms	N/A	1 tbsp	2tbsp	3 tbsp
strawberries	3	4	6	6-8
sweetcorn kernels	1 tbsp	2 tbsp	2 tbsp	3 tbsp
tinned or frozen fruit	1/2 tbsp	1 tbsp	2 tbsp	3 tbsp

Portion sizes are approximate – size and weight of your child should also be taken into consideration.

These supplements, manufactured specifically for children, contain natural foods including brown rice, carrot juice, spinach and broccoli in a tropical flavoured chewy tablet.

Probiotics (friendly bacteria) for children are also available as supplements. The right balance of bacteria is vital for good health but often neglected or forgotten. Without the good bacteria, however, nutrients in food and other supplements are simply not absorbed effectively. Probiotics can be especially helpful for children who have repeatedly been given antibiotics. In addition to fighting bacteria that might cause the infection, antibiotics also damage and deplete good bacteria in the gut that is essential for effective digestion and strong immunity. Symptoms of deficiency may include poor concentration, constant fatigue, recurrent infections such as colds and digestive or skin problems. Probiotic drinks and yogurts usually contain sugar and low levels of beneficial bacteria. Children also require good bacteria that are different from those that adults need – it is therefore a good idea to buy probiotics that are especially produced for children. These can be purchased from health food shops or online but it is best to consult a registered nutritionist first to discuss the alternatives.

Single supplements such as vitamin C are available separately and this can be useful in addition to a multivitamin and mineral if fighting off an infection.

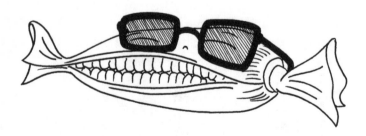

Which ones?

With the wide range of supplements available it can be confusing for parents – are some brands better than others for example and in what forms and doses can they be given for different age groups? It is best to give supplements that are specifically for children, but as a rough guide –

- 4-6 years – one quarter of an adult dose
- 7-10 years – half of an adult dose
- 11-14 years – three quarters of an adult dose
- 15 + years equivalent to an adult dose

Avoid brands that are flavoured with sugar or sweeteners or that have artificial additives and flavouring. Also try to ensure that they have high enough levels for the age of your child. The official RDA* and RNI* levels set by the health department are high enough to prevent disease and deficiency but some nutrients that are included may not be at a level to ensure optimum health. With supplements it really is the case that you get what you pay for, and that cheaper brands may contain low levels of nutrients of perhaps inferior quality that, although it may be better than taking no supplements at all, might not be very well absorbed.

The best supplements tend to be those sold in health food shops or through natural health web sites and mail order, produced by companies that specialise in supplement manufacture. These are more likely to have optimum levels of nutrients, be especially formulated for children, be sugar free, have natural flavouring and be free from additives and animal products. Never give more than the recommended dose of any supplement to children – always read labels carefully.

*RDA = Recommended Daily Allowance
*RNI = Reference Nutrient Intakes

Getting them down

Some supplements are available in drops, liquid or powder form that can be mixed with drinks or disguised in food. If supplements taste pleasant, children over four may be happy to suck or chew tablets, but do ensure that you keep them out of reach – young children may mistake them for sweets and very high levels of some nutrients can be toxic.

Omega oils can be difficult to disguise but come in various flavoured preparations that have an acceptable, if not pleasant, taste. Small amounts can also be added to milkshakes or juice.

A list of supplement suppliers is given on the White Ladder web site – **www.whiteladderpress.com**

2

Hiding vegetables and other good stuff

Many parents say that vegetables are often left on their child's plate if served with a family meal. If the same goes for you, this chapter might help.

If vegetables are served separately and your child prefers other things on the plate, it is understandable that they might eat what they feel like and leave the vegetables. However, if the vegetables are mixed in with the food they like, it is possible to get everything down at once with minimum effort.

Most vegetables can be disguised to blend in with other food, but follow these five tips for a better chance of success:

Tip One – Choose your colours carefully

Trying to blend broccoli into mashed potato, for example, will not work well. Kids are suspicious of 'bits', especially 'green bits' and try as you might it won't disappear. Half a parsnip or a little cauliflower, boiled and mashed with the potato (perhaps with added cheese to disguise the taste) will look and taste fine.

Similarly, apple can't be easily hidden in chocolate cake, but prunes (dried or tinned) can be blended in perfectly.

Tip Two – Don't leave lumps

Children can be particularly unforgiving when it comes to lumps in their food. If they find one small lump they will probably leave the whole lot, and refuse to eat that dish for a very long time, if ever again. Cook, mash and blend the food properly to avoid this problem. If you don't have a blender or food processor it is worth investing in one to save your arm if nothing else. A case of 'mashing shoulder' or 'whisking wrist' can feel much worse if the food you prepare is left anyway.

Tip Three – Add just a little

Don't go in for overkill when adding vegetables to meals and fruit to puddings or you may spoil the taste and your effort will be wasted. Go for the drip feed effect with added goodness – a little every day will have a cumulative effect and will be beneficial in the long term. As a rough guide, replace one tenth of the usual ingredients with vegetable or fruit to begin with and blend in well. For example, replace part of a pasta meat sauce with finely chopped vegetables. See how this works and if the children eat it without comment you can always add a little more next time.

Tip Four – Introduce changes slowly

Try a home cooked meal with well hidden vegetables around once a week to begin with, working up to several meals a week over a few months. If you suddenly become a home cooking super mum or dad, kids are likely to rebel. Gradually get used to adding a little something to all their meals, even if it is just a sprinkling of herbs, some vegetable water in the gravy or a spoonful of peas with their fish fingers and chips.

Tip Five – Start with food you know they like

If your children rarely eat shepherd's pie, it isn't a good idea to start by hiding vegetables in this. Think about things you know they like – pizza maybe – and work out ways to make it a little healthier, perhaps by adding blended or finely chopped vegetables to the topping.

What to hide and how to hide it

Vegetables

Bean sprouts are obviously great in stir-fries or added to rice or noodles. They can also be shredded (preferably in a blender) and added to home made burgers.

Beans and pulses are soft and have a mild flavour so can be added, whole or mashed, to any dish such as soups, shepherd's pie, burgers or curry.

Broccoli Boiled in a little water or steamed, broccoli becomes very soft and easy to mash for adding to home made burgers, pasta sauce or pizza topping (but don't overdo it as lots of green does not look appetising). Leftovers can be used in bubble and squeak. Equally good as small, crunchy florets in stir-fry.

Cabbage/Sprouts Not often a favourite with children but if chosen well (young and sweet) and cooked properly (not too soggy and with a little butter) your child may develop a taste for these vegetables. They are not easily disguised but shredded cabbage can be stir-fried and both can be used in bubble and squeak.

Carrots Grated carrot can be added to cakes and puddings before cooking as it is naturally sweet. Boiled and mashed or finely chopped and fried it can be added to pasta sauce, pizza topping, soup, stew, shepherd's pie, curry and home made burgers (see also 'orange mash', below). Shredded or finely chopped sticks add colour to stir-fries and salads.

Cauliflower With the great advantage of being white and also very soft when cooked, this vegetable can be hidden in places that other vegetables cannot reach. It mashes in with potato or blends with cheese sauce perfectly. It can also be stir-fried and the old favourite, cauliflower cheese, is still a hit with many kids (with fried onions, a little garlic and lots of cheese, served with a side vegetable or two, it takes care of several portions all in one go).

Courgette These are baby marrows that have a taste that is different from the fully grown version. Use grated or mashed in soups, sauces and stir-fries or even thinly sliced on top of pizza.

Garlic crushed or finely chopped and fried adds a lovely subtle flavour to pasta sauce, bolognaise sauce, pizza topping, soup, stew, shepherd's pie, stir-fry and curry.

Herbs A wide variety of herbs can be purchased at supermarkets and if growing in pots they are fresh until used. Better still, grow your own in the garden or in pots in your kitchen. Add a handful of chopped herbs to any savoury dish or use as a garnish. Dried or frozen herbs work well in cooking too.

Mange-tout work well in stir-fries and salads.

Mushrooms High in protein and a useful addition to the diet if your child does not eat meat. Mushrooms can be chopped and added to home made burgers, curry, pasta sauce, soup, stew and shepherd's pie. Sliced mushrooms can be stir-fried or used as a pizza topping.

Onions finely chopped and gently fried in pasta sauce, curry, pizza topping, home made burgers, soup, stew and shepherd's pie. Slices or rings, gently fried in olive oil, make a tasty garnish for hot dogs or burgers. Raw onion rings, brushed with olive oil, can be added to pizza topping before baking or grilling.

Parsnip boiled and mashed with potato becomes almost invisible. Chopped into small pieces, parsnip can be added to soups and stews and it can also be roasted in chunks or wedges as a change from potato.

Peas Petits pois are best as they are sweeter and softer than fully grown peas. Add to rice, shepherd's pie and curry or mash into home made burgers.

Peppers are an acquired taste for some, so introduce them slowly and in small amounts. Chopped and fried they can be added to curry, pizza topping, pasta sauce and soup. Finely shredded they add taste and variety to stir-fries and salads.

Pumpkin or squash These can be used in sweet or savoury dishes. Pumpkin soup is a great autumn and winter warmer – getting kids to choose or even grow their own may encourage them to try eating them too. Chopped into other soups and stews they turn soft and add flavour. Sweet pumpkin pie with cream or ice cream makes a different dessert.

Runner beans or green beans should be young, not stringy. They can be finely chopped and added to sauces, soups and stews.

Swede Many children actually like the taste of raw swede as a salad vegetable. If not it can be boiled and mashed with a little butter on its own or with other vegetables.

Sweet Potato A lovely flavour with more vitamins and fibre than ordinary potato – makes great roasted wedges and can be used as a substitute wherever you would normally use potato.

Sweetcorn Kernels can be added to pizza topping or rice, and baby corn is great in stir-fry or as a side vegetable. Corn-on-the-cob is loved by most kids either steamed, baked or barbecued (wrap in foil with a little butter before cooking).

Tomatoes The most versatile of vegetables (although, yes, it's really a fruit) and also extremely nutritious, you can use fresh or tinned tomatoes in a wide variety of food. Chopped or blended, boiled or fried, as liquid or reduced to a paste (by slowly boiling off the excess liquid), tomato can be used in pasta sauce, pizza topping, soup, stew, shepherd's pie, curry and home made burgers. Making your own ketchup just now and again is well worth the effort. Try home made tomato soup too – it has less salt and sugar than the tinned variety and will be higher in nutrients. Keep a tube of tomato purée in the fridge, ready to squeeze into all sorts of dishes.

Fruit

Apple & pear When stewed these can be served with rice pudding, custard or even ice cream for a different dessert. Grated or finely chopped apple or pear can be added to cake mix before baking or pancake mixture before cooking.

Apricots Lovely and sweet, fresh apricots can be added to yoghurt and fruit salad, purées or sorbets and make nice jam, Dried they can be finely chopped and added to cakes and puddings.

Bananas Versatile and packed with nutrients, you no longer need to suffer squashed, blackened bananas at the bottom of your child's lunch box. Bananas can be mashed and used as sandwich filling, chopped in a fruit salad or blended into cake mix before baking. Banana split is a fun dessert that most children love.

Grapes Small, sweet and seedless they are lovely in a fruit salad or on their own.

Kiwi fruit Packed with vitamin C, make sure they are well ripened and add to yoghurt and fruit salad or blend into smoothies.

Mango Once tasted, your children will love this sweet, soft, tropical fruit. Make sure they are well ripened but not overripe, cut out the stone and serve in slices, chopped in yogurt or added to fruit salad. Mangoes also make wonderful smoothies.

Oranges & Lemons Use the zest, grated into cakes and puddings (but wash them well first), and use the juice in drinks or to make ice cubes.

Pineapple Fresh or canned, they are sweet and nutritious. Add chunks to fruit salad, use the juice in drinks and ice cubes and add crushed pineapple to yogurt, smoothies, cakes and puddings.

Plums make lovely, low sugar jam to last all year. Stew and have with milk puddings and leave plenty in the fruit bowl for snacking.

Prunes Dried or tinned in juice, prunes can be stewed and added to puddings or blended in cakes – and they have the great advantage of being the same colour as chocolate...

Raisins Great on their own as a snack, they can also be added to cakes, scones, milk puddings and sprinkled on cereals.

Raspberries Mostly the same as for strawberries, **but** younger children may find raspberry pips a little troublesome. If this is a problem, mash or purée and then strain though a sieve.

Strawberries Although most children like strawberries anyway, they can also be puréed and added to milkshakes, smoothies and sorbets or chopped in fruit salad and yoghurt or on cereal. You can even make your own jam using more fruit and pectin with less sugar (yes, it is a fag but once a year can give you months of supplies).

Parent-to-parent ideas, tips and tricks

Almost every parent has at least one way of getting their child to eat fruit and vegetables, from plain old bribery to far more sneaky measures.

Here is a selection of the best ideas, gathered from nutritionists and chefs but mostly from ordinary parents:

Wait until they have visitors

The best time to try something new is when your children have friends over for a meal. Whether it is a main course with well hidden vegetables or a pudding consisting mainly of fruit, the friends will not know that this is different from the norm. If other children eat the food without question, yours should too. Don't hover, watch or comment – just serve the food and disappear.

Peel and chop fruit for them

Children, lovely as they are, can be lazy when it comes to eating. Whether it is peeling an orange or chewing their way through a whole apple (including skin), usually they just can't be bothered. For pudding, snacks or supper, they are much more likely to eat fruit if you do the hard work. Serve it immediately after preparation – brown apples and soggy strawberries are not appetising.

You could include:

• Peeled bananas, chopped into chunks

• A couple of peeled and segmented satsumas

• A few strawberries, washed, dried and without the stalks

• A handful of grapes, washed and dried

• An apple or pear, peeled and chopped

• Some cherries, washed and dried without the stalks (removing the stones is a little extreme, unless your children are young enough to choke on them)

• Sweet oranges, cut into quarters or eighths with the skin on – children love to suck the juice whilst making funny faces with the orange skin over their teeth

• Small, ripe apricots, washed, cut in half with stones removed

• Kiwi fruit – peeled and sliced or cut into quarters, or halved so they can be scooped out and eaten with a teaspoon

• Slices of mango, papaya, and pineapple add a tropical taste for a refreshing change

Start with one

If your child says that they do not like a certain vegetable, maybe they don't, but maybe they have not even tried it. When serving the vegetable with a family meal, put just one (or one teaspoon) of this vegetable on their plate – yes, even one pea. If they comment, pretend that it slipped onto the plate 'by mistake'. You may need to do this several times before they eat it, but before you know it they may be asking for more.

Bargaining

Make a meal with three types of vegetable. If they complain or attempt to leave them all, make out you are doing them a favour by letting them leave two if they eat one.

If they protest that they don't want to try vegetables or fruit, agree with them that if they try something 10 times and still don't like it they will not have to eat it again.

Get them to count

Explain to your children about the health benefits of fruit and vegetables – their school should be reinforcing this as part of the curriculum. At the end of the day (just occasionally, not every day) ask them in the evening how many portions of fruit and vegetables they have eaten that day. Praise them or give a small reward (a gold star, 10p) if they have had five or over. The Rainbow Food Activity Chart can help with this (see The benefits of fruit and vegetables, chapter one).

Bribe them!

Not every parent agrees with bribery, but you may find it works and it can help in the short term to get them used to new foods. Offer them something as a reward for eating up all their vegetables or finishing a plate of fruit, but not every day or every mealtime. The danger is they will expect rewards for eating vegetables, even when they get older. A new bike or a holiday with friends is no fair exchange for your teenager eating their carrots…

Disguise with cheese

If your child likes cheese, and most do, try vegetables in cheese sauce (broccoli, cauliflower, onions, garlic etc) or grated cheese, melted if preferred, over the top.

Fondue!

Have fun with a savoury sauce like cheese or spicy tomato and either raw or very lightly cooked vegetables. Similarly, a sweet or chocolate sauce can help a whole load of fruit go down without any problem.

Use the water

Always try to save the water in which you cook your green vegetables. Lots of vitamins leak into the water when the vegetables are cooking and rather than throwing this away, use it to make gravy or add to soup and stew.

Salad

Start adding a little salad to finger food – sandwiches, chips, pizza or nuggets. Just two or three chunky cucumber slices, a cherry tomato or two and a few little carrot sticks can make quite a difference to the nutritional content of a child's meal or snack. Don't comment if they leave some but give the same amount each time – the amount that they eat should gradually increase.

Stir-fry

Many children love beansprouts, not least because they look like worms. Stir-fry for just a couple of minutes (not until they go soggy) with finely sliced carrots, peppers and onions and serve with rice or noodles. Speaking of rice, add chopped herbs, finely chopped onions, peas and sweetcorn to your fried rice – delicious!

Call it something interesting

Young children can be persuaded to try almost anything if they like the sound of it. Pirate's pie, fairy swirl, fisherman's lunch, giant's mountains, princess picnic, etc.

Orange mash

Instead of boring mashed potato with their sausages or on top of shepherd's pie, make the mash orange with carrots, swede and sweet potato – it looks and tastes more interesting and a little cheese can be added to improve the taste.

Garnish everything

Whether you grow your own on the kitchen windowsill or buy them fresh or growing in pots, a sprinkling of finely chopped herbs in every savoury dish can contribute to the daily intake of vitamins. Most have a subtle flavour and your children will soon get so used to seeing a garnish they will not even notice after a while.

Roast everything

Don't just stick to roast potatoes with your roast dinner. Roasting carrots, peppers, onions, sweet potatoes, parsnips, tomatoes, mushrooms and baby sweetcorn can make a great meal with minimum meat.

Batter it

A simple batter can transform dull food into an exciting snack. Cut fruit or vegetables into bite-size pieces and dip into batter mix, then fry in olive oil or butter. Serve battered vegetables with salsa, mayonnaise or ketchup and battered fruit with honey, puréed fruit or melted chocolate.

Grow your own

If you have a garden and just a little time, growing your own fruit and vegetables with the help of your children will not only educate them about where food comes from but encourage them to eat what they grow. It is much more interesting for children to eat peas they have picked and shelled for dinner or to take an apple picked from a tree in their own garden in their school lunch box. Even if you don't have a garden, a few herbs or small fruits (eg strawberries) can be grown in pots. Children also love growing their own cress from seed in little pots with cotton wool at the bottom.

Go picking

If you don't have room in your garden to grow fruit or vegetables, or don't have the time or inclination, pick-your-own is a good alternative.

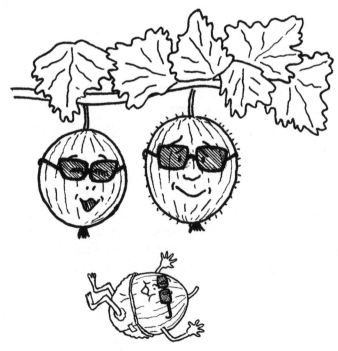

Farms and market gardens everywhere use pick-your-own as a way to offer cheaper produce and also save on labour costs. Make an outing to pick strawberries and take a picnic to have with them afterwards – this is an enjoyable and cheap day out. Vegetable picking too can be interesting for young children, especially if they are allowed to wash and prepare them at home for eating or freezing. Label them with the child's name 'Lizzie's peas, September 2004' or 'Jake's raspberries, July 2005' – this will not only remind them of a nice day out but encourage them to eat up when they are served.

Cheat with baby food

If your child is averse to lumps, jars of baby food are a great way to add nutritious ingredients to many dishes. They are also now low in salt and sugar and many contain just puréed fruit or vegetables. Add vegetable baby food to soup and sauces – fruit baby food can be added to yogurt, cream, custard or ice cream.

3

Habits and psychology

Breaking old habits

It isn't going to be easy making changes to the food your children eat and even the most careful, patient parent will probably find that the little ones will rebel at some point and to some degree.

The problem is, many of us learned about eating food that is good for us the hard way and the temptation is to continue with these parental habits with our own children.

If you were made to sit at the table until you had cleaned your plate you are not alone – most of the adult population have suffered this at some point, at school if not at home. Forcing your child to eat, especially if they don't like what is on the plate, is completely counterproductive. 'Sit there until you finish' may be how we learned, and the only way you feel able to achieve your agenda, but think about it – the experience of eating a pile of unwanted cabbage until they feel sick is hardly going to make a child jump for joy the next time it is served. Also, many adults who now battle to keep their weight healthy suffer from having been conditioned to finish everything on their plate even if they neither want nor need it. As obesity problems increase, this isn't a helpful legacy to pass on to our children.

This heavy handed approach is so last century and you may win the battle but you definitely won't win the war. Most children, like most adults, have something they don't like the taste of – try to respect this and avoid giving them things to eat that they don't like.

Withholding puddings used to be thought of as a good idea too, but guess what? That doesn't work either. 'No pudding until you have finished your main course' was the standard line when most parents of today were young and is still commonly used, but only makes sweet things seem more desirable.

Children can quickly learn to use food as a weapon against you if they discover that you are easily stressed or upset by what they do or don't eat. Remember there is a world of difference between force and encouragement. Try to put your child into a position where they want to eat well and enjoy their food, rather than eating food or being deprived of treats as punishment.

Set an example

The habit of eating as a family is disappearing, the result being the loss of parents as role models. Family mealtimes have largely been replaced by different eating times and different menus.

It can be extremely difficult for working parents to arrange a sit down meal daily for the whole family. School, work and leisure timetables during the week can often mean a meal for children in the afternoon with adults eating much later in the evening, often when children are in bed.

In a two parent family, the adults may like to eat in peace or one might wait until the other returns from work so that they can eat together – this can often be the only time that parents have the opportunity to be together without the children. If this is important to you and you feel reluctant to give this up, the stay-at-home parent could eat twice. This is not to suggest that two full sized portions of dinner are consumed on a regular basis as this might not do a lot for your waistline. However, the concept of 'little and often' is thought to be healthier and a token small plate of food just to keep the children or your partner company can do no harm.

If you are a lone parent it can be tempting to eat alone as it is often less stressful. Sitting down to eat with the children, however, will encourage them into good habits, but only, of course, if you eat healthily too. When children see that eating fruit and vegetables is the normal thing to do they are much more likely to continue this habit, even when you are not there to keep an eye on them.

When the family does eat together, try to create habit and ritual that they can join in with – praise them if they help to lay the table and give them responsibility for one task, even a small one, to help them feel that they are making a contribution to the mealtime. If the family can eat together only occasionally, and you have more than one set of crockery or cutlery, make one your 'best' set, only for use at family mealtimes. Allowing children to use grown-up cups or glasses will also make them feel important and more likely to copy you in other ways too – even eating sprouts.

Take care also with the type of food that you eat in the presence of your children. If they see you eating chips, burgers, cake, biscuits, pies etc they are likely, even subconsciously, to copy you. Eat your vegetables with relish (including 'mmm, delicious' sound effects) have apples and bananas for snacks, eat fruit puddings and add salad to your sandwiches (you can scoff the chips and chocolate when they are in bed).

Give praise

Children usually respond well to praise so don't miss the opportunity when they do eat well to praise them for it. Praise can help improve any difficult situation and eating well is no different. The feel-good factor of a pleased mum or dad, a smile and nice comment can go a long way. Children don't usually want to be difficult, they just want attention – bad attention (shouting, smacks, criticism) is sometimes better than none, but good attention is a whole lot better. Children who are eager to please and want to maintain the approval of their parents are not only happier but easier to manage.

Talk about it

Explain to your children from an early age that vegetables and fruit are important for their health and growth. Initiate conversation about their diet and point out that they are able to do the things that they like if they eat well. Sporty children may be encouraged by being told that a good diet is essential for energy and a well functioning body. It can also do no harm to suggest that their favourite sports star obviously eats lots of fruit and vegetables to stay fit and strong. The more sedentary child also needs the essential nutrients gained from a good diet to stay well and fight off infections. Even computer or playstation addicts can benefit from a good diet to stay alert, maintain sharp eyesight and improve quick reflexes.

Rather than giving no choice to children about what they eat, ask them what they like and dislike, what they might want for dinner in the coming week or what they might like you to buy when you go shopping. If they ask for pizza, explain that this is fine but that they do need to eat vegetables or salad with it and ask what they would prefer. Try to show the same consideration as you would for another adult and this will hopefully result in less conflict over food.

Understand, don't fight

Avoid arguing or becoming angry with your children over food at all costs. If mealtimes have become a battle, try stepping back and adopting a more easygoing attitude. Bite your tongue and grit your teeth for a while, even if they will only eat chocolate pudding. Trust that they will soon become tired of it and will ask for a proper meal before too long.

Children do have reasons for developing food fads and they do not necessarily have control over this. For example, a research study on hunter-gatherers (which we all were until a few thousand years ago) showed that once children become mobile they will instinctively become fussier about the food that they will eat. This is thought to be a protective mechanism as once away from a parent, the child might accidentally eat something poisonous. Therefore, the subconscious will restrict the food that a toddler will eat so that they will stick to things that are familiar and safe.

Another theory on human preference explains why we are attracted to sweet or high calorie food. Before supermarkets and instant snacks, food was often in short supply. We are genetically programmed to like this food because it was important in our past for people to eat when they could, as a regular supply of food could not be guaranteed. Stocking up on calories was an essential safeguard for times when food was scarce.

Remember also that children have smaller bodies and smaller stomachs, so will not physically be able to eat as much as you might like them to. Three square meals a day is enough for most adults, but children need to eat more often in order to maintain stable blood sugar levels. If you try to fit children into your pattern of eating, and restrict or forbid any snacking between main meals, this may result in moods and tantrums that they have little control over. Five or six smaller meals and snacks can maintain blood sugar levels and help to ensure an even mood.

'Use it or lose it' is a well known saying and is actually a proven fact in this context – humans are creatures of habit and usually stick with what they are familiar with. Once any habit, including eating junk food, is established, the brain actually wires up to this way of thinking. For example, taking sugar in your tea, going round the supermarket shelves the same way, having fish on a Friday are habits that, once fixed in your brain can be difficult to change. This is because your brain has to rewire to another way of thinking, and can only do this by repetitive practice.

Don't be surprised, therefore, if your children can't get out of the chicken nugget habit all at once and 'forget' or rebel against having vegetables more often. Anyone who has given up sugar in tea will know that after a while the new way seems the only way – accidentally drinking tea with sugar in can make you gag. Having fruit for pudding or fresh herbs sprinkled on a main meal may take a little getting used to, but given time will seem perfectly normal and should not be questioned.

Giving them choice

Adults like to feel that they are in control of their children, however this is achieved, but children also like to feel that they have choices, even if these are limited.

If you can cope with children helping to shop and prepare food this is an excellent way to give children some choice and make them feel important. Asking 'what vegetables shall we buy this week?' and allowing them to select, place in the bag and take to the checkout will give them a feeling of ownership. Talk about 'your lovely carrots' or 'that nice broccoli you chose' and they will be far more likely to eat it when mealtime comes.

If you have more than one child let them take turns in coming to the supermarket with you or ask one child to choose the vegetables and another one the fruit, for example.

Taking this idea one step further, growing a few fruit or vegetables in the garden means that children can feel that they have not only chosen the food but created it. Start by shopping for seeds, letting them choose what they want to grow, plant them together and let children help with watering and picking. If you don't have enough space, a few pots can hold small fruit or a selection of herbs.

Unless you are a super calm parent or on medication, allowing children to help with food preparation can be a stressful business. Being allowed to help just occasionally, however, can help your child to feel that they are contributing to the food that they eat.

Even if there are limited choices, asking children for their preferences can make it harder for them to refuse the food when it is served. 'Would you prefer sweetcorn or peas today?' might seem a pointless question and it is just easier to cook whatever you think best, but it can be important to the child and when presented with their choice they may be less likely to leave it.

Just for you

Indulging your children for a short time, just while they get used to new tastes, can help establish good new habits. If they are reluctant to try things, getting smaller versions or making smaller portions 'just for you' may help them to feel special and make them more inclined to taste something new. Pick out the smallest strawberries and put on to a saucer with a sprinkling of sugar, select mini-sized fruit for their lunch box or picnic, buy petits pois, baby sweetcorn, button mushrooms, the smallest, sweetest carrots or make individual child sized cakes or savoury pies. Once vegetables and fruit are an established part of their diet you can slowly phase this out and serve normal portions.

Make it fun

Turning food time into fun occasionally can make eating healthy food enjoyable.

- Making a picnic, even to eat in the garden or local park, is far more interesting than sitting in the same old kitchen. (The added bonus of a picnic away from home is that you have a captive audience that has little choice but to eat the food that is on offer or go hungry. Oh dear, you forgot the crisps but brought cucumber chunks instead. If chocolate bars have been left behind there is always a banana, and what a shame – you accidentally put lettuce in their sandwiches too. Stay for the whole day and your children will be less fussy as they become hungrier.)

- If the weather is wet or cold, suggest an indoor picnic on the living room floor (with a sheet to catch the crumbs). Better still, pack a container of 'rations' in a napkin and get them to pretend that they are on an adventure – deep in the jungle, climbing a mountain or crossing a desert (where there is no kitchen with chocolate biscuits or lemonade for miles).

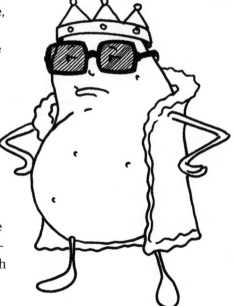

- Another game that children love is 'restaurants'. It takes some planning but is worth it, even if you are only able to manage it occasionally. Draw up a menu with selections for starters, main meal, choice of vegetables and dessert (making sure that each option has some-thing healthy). Set the table with folded napkins and get them to come in to the dining room, take their coats and call them 'sir' or 'madam'. Wear an apron or drape a tea towel over your arm, pour their fruit juice into glasses and ask them to 'enjoy your meal' when served. They will feel so important and grown–up that they are almost sure to eat everything. When you do actually eat out, suggest that they are 'too grown-up' for the kiddies menu and instead order a small portion of an adult meal.

4

Saving time and effort

When stay-at-home mums had all the time in the world, home cooked food was the norm and patience was in much greater supply than for most busy working parents of today.

Growing fresh vegetables in the garden, shopping with the children, making cakes with them and playing 'adventures' or 'restaurants' are literally impossible to fit in to most busy families more than very occasionally, if at all.

All the planning and time management in the world cannot double the amount of time you have or enable you to be in two places at once. First of all, don't feel guilty about not doing it all – there are not enough hours in the day to do the many jobs that parents need to do. Second, get help if you need it, even if you have to pay someone.

If your work is as a homemaker, although modern gadgets do make some tasks easier there may be more demands on your time than the housewife of 40 years ago. They were probably not expected to contribute to the family income, would not have been encouraged to further their education, were not asked to help out at school and often didn't have much of a social life. Their role was defined as housekeeper and childminder – full stop (and it was almost always mum that stayed at home in the past, whereas now more dads than ever are taking on the role).

Once a year

If the mention of baking cakes, making jam, taking a picnic with the children or growing vegetables are things that leave you cold or fill you with dread, resolving to do something once a year may make it seem manageable. Don't feel that you should be making cakes every week or taking picnics every weekend throughout the summer, just try to do things like this once a year. This way you may actually enjoy it.

Going to pick fruit at the local farm can be made into an afternoon out that keeps the children occupied and doesn't cost much. Making cakes at home with the children, even if only for the summer fête or Christmas draw, can be satisfying and rewarding (for the children if not for you), and growing one pot of herbs or a few tomatoes each year still gives children the experience without wearing you out too much.

Some tasks, such as making jam or freezing fresh vegetables, have a long lasting benefit that can give you a feeling of satisfaction even weeks or months later.

Save time preparing meals

- Food processors, blenders and electric mixers can take so much effort out of food preparation whether it is chopping, grating or mixing more thoroughly than you ever could. If you are preparing something that you use often you can chop double and keep half in a lidded container or food bag in the fridge for the next day.

- Some vegetables, broccoli for example, can be chopped up and stalks discarded all in one go and the individual florets kept in the fridge to use when you are ready.

- If you are a very busy parent, and can afford it, buy bags of vegetables ready to use – chopped and washed – from the supermarket. You could also keep a couple of bags of frozen vegetables as a standby.

- Jars of garlic and ginger, finely chopped or minced, are available from many supermarkets but need to be kept in the fridge and used within a certain time once you have opened them.

- Garlic purée is also a good standby if you are short of time.

- If you don't have the inclination to grow herbs in pots on the kitchen windowsill, fresh herbs growing in pots are now widely available in supermarkets.

- If you can't be bothered to get out the kitchen scales (and wash them up afterwards), it is handy to know that a rounded tablespoon of flour equals roughly one ounce and a level tablespoon of sugar equals about one ounce.

Plan ahead

It can be difficult to think about the evening meal at the start of a busy day but planning ahead can save time and effort later on. Friday's dinner might not be the first thing on your mind when you are shopping days beforehand but making a weekly menu can save time, reduce stress and make everyone in the household happier about what they eat. Spend a few minutes thinking about meals for the week ahead and then write a shopping list for everything you will need.

If you can, involve the children in planning the weekly menu. This may involve some bargaining 'we can have pizza if we eat fruit for pudding' or 'jelly is OK for dessert if we have chicken and three vegetables for main course'. This may get children used to the idea that at every mealtime there should be at least some fruit or vegetable content. There will be occasions when flexibility is required – an extra little mouth or two to feed for example – so swap the meals around or keep one meal for another day and do something quick instead (like go to the chip shop).

With your weekly menu on display on the fridge or kitchen notice board, when you get up in the morning you can start preparing for the evening meal without effort. Take chicken breasts or mince out of the freezer first thing in the morning, peel potatoes or chop a few vegetables at lunchtime or as soon as you get in from work and half the preparation is already done. It may seem a small thing, but a loud, persistent kitchen timer is a must for any busy parent who cooks, and will save you from burnt offerings and blackened saucepans.

Forward planning isn't just good for cooking meals, but can be used in any situation where children need to eat. Packing lunch-boxes with all but the fresh food at night will mean less rush and effort in the morning. Thinking about a family picnic the day before you go allows time for shopping and preparation. You can even prepare for eating out by checking out menus in advance.

Shopping wisely

Once you have your weekly menu, shopping should become easier and faster than just browsing around the shelves. Buy plenty of healthier snacks too (see snacks, part two) and gradually you can conveniently forget to buy chocolate biscuits and other less healthy snacks. Plan too for lunchboxes each day, and add everything you will need to your list.

If possible, shop alone except as an occasional treat for the kids so that you are not persuaded to buy sweets and treats.

Internet shopping can be an absolute godsend for many busy parents, but if you spend all day at your computer it can actually be an enjoyable outing when you go out to the supermarket (sad, but true). If you do shop online, it may take hours the first time you try it – this might leave you wondering why you bothered and make you seriously question the advantages. Once you are practised, however, the friendly computer remembers everything you have bought before (and everything you usually buy in the local store, if you use a loyalty card). You then have the option of selecting your favourites each time and your weekly shopping can be done in 14 minutes flat at 11pm from the comfort of your living room. Supermarkets are very keen to promote this method of shopping (maybe because it keeps the pesky customers away) and competition is fierce, so you may find that there are generous incentives. Although there is generally a delivery charge, this is usually more than saved by the lack of browsing and impulse buying, and more than worth it to save fatigue and frayed nerves.

Make the most of your freezer

It is wonderfully satisfying to come home after a busy day and take a home made meal from the freezer to heat and eat. This can be a reality at least once a week if you follow this simple rule – every time you cook something at home, make double or treble and freeze the remainder. Invest in some freezer-to-microwave containers with airtight lids for home made soups or sauces for bolognaise and curry. Cook the whole amount of sauce or soup, cool the half for freezing completely and pour into the container, seal securely then freeze on the same day that it has been cooked.

There are many other ways that a freezer can save you time and effort:

• Make a large batch of cakes and freeze half.

• Fresh fruit sorbet frozen in small tubs makes an instant dessert.

• Fresh herbs can be chopped and frozen in small containers or even an ice cube tray for a last minute addition to your cooking.

- Fresh fruit juice can be made into ice cubes or lollies (see puddings and sweet treats).

- Freeze stewed fruit or home made fruit pies for making a quick pudding.

- Vegetables that have been ready washed and partly cooked can save you time when you are in a hurry – you can do this yourself or buy them ready prepared.

- Some supermarkets, health food shops and farms sell ready made frozen organic meals to use as an occasional standby.

Your freezer can help you to save time in lots of ways, even if the only vegetable you keep in it is a bag of frozen peas.

Help with school packed lunches

Making a packed lunch for children every day can be a drag, especially if you make one for yourself or your spouse as well. Whilst some items can be packed the night before or grabbed from the freezer or cupboard (see packed lunches, part two) it still requires imagination and commitment to make a lunchbox healthy day after day.

You can buy ready packed healthier lunches for children in some areas from catering businesses or specialist services that deliver to schools, such as this one that operates in Surrey and is expanding into London – **www.lunchboxes4kids.com** (This company, run by a husband and wife team, is hoping to launch franchise businesses throughout the country, so contact them if you would like to work for yourself and help local children to eat healthier packed lunches.)

School lunches may seem an easy option and they can also work out cheaper, but they are not always as nutritious as they could be, although in some areas this is improving. School meals must offer at least one portion of fruit and one portion of vegetables each day, in addition to one dairy item, one portion of protein source and a portion of starchy food. The key word here is 'offer'. Local authority catering departments can offer vegetables as a side dish and fruit as a dessert, but that doesn't mean that children will choose them – almost every child would go for an iced bun rather than a banana or apple.

If you do opt for school lunches, ask your school to show you menus. You can look at them with your children to get an idea of the choices they are likely to make. If you don't feel that the food on offer is healthy enough or offers enough choice, speak to the school or local authority catering department. Ask your children each day (casually, of course) what they had for lunch, just as you ask them what lessons they had or who they played with. If their answers are consistently along the lines of 'chicken teddies and chips with chocolate cake for pudding', question the school about their policy on encouraging children towards the healthier choices.

Changes and additions to fast food

Busy parents will sometimes need to rely on convenience food for their children. When you are extra busy, tired, ill, haven't been able to get to the supermarket or are just completely whacked, how can you make an average tea time a little bit healthier?

- Give fish fingers, burgers or chicken nuggets but cook frozen vegetables to go with them.

- Add chopped fresh herbs to tinned soup.

- Make or buy a fast food snack or meal but serve with fruit juice.

- Put thinly sliced cucumber, grated carrot or cress in sandwiches.

- Serve fruit for pudding, even if it is tinned.

- Beans on toast counts as one portion. Make the toast wholemeal and add tomato purée and chopped fresh or dried herbs to the beans.

- Make bolognaise with sauce from a jar but with fried onions, extra tomatoes and chopped fresh herbs.

- Similarly, use curry sauce in a jar but add chopped vegetables to the onions when frying before you add the meat or chicken. Add a few frozen peas to the rice when it is cooking.

- Get fish and chips in an emergency but serve with peas or cucumber slices sprinkled with grated carrot and cress. Ketchup has healthy ingredients but can also contain quite high levels of sugar and salt.

- Buy ready made fresh soup, blend if necessary to eliminate 'lumps and bits', and warm in a saucepan with a sprinkling of herbs.

- Cook a ready made pizza with potato wedges instead of chips and serve with salad sticks and dips.

- Make a quick omelette with some chopped onion, mushrooms and tomato fried together before adding the egg mixture.

- Serve quick sausage and bean casserole (see children's meals in part two).

Ten things you can do right now, without effort, to improve the health of your family

If many of the ideas in other chapters sound daunting or you really don't have the time, here are 10 improvements that you can make to your family diet. Although they will not increase your child's intake of fruit and vegetables, these simple measures may at least help make your household healthier. All can be managed with little effort or expense.

1 Change fizzy drinks to high juice squash or fruit juice (one glass of fruit juice counts towards one portion a day). Add sparkling mineral water for a fizzy drink.

Why? Soft carbonated drinks contain chemicals, encourage sweet tooth, can damage bones if intake is prolonged and contribute to obesity.

2 Use filtered water for cooking, drinking, diluting squash and making ice cubes. Filter jugs cost just a few pounds – keep topped up in the fridge and remember to change the cartridge monthly.

Why? Filtering water before drinking helps to remove chemicals and toxins.

3 Change from ordinary salt to low sodium salt for all cooking and table use. LoSalt and Solo are widely available in supermarkets.

Why? Salt is present in many processed foods and most people consume far more than is healthy for them. High salt intake can damage kidneys and lead to high blood pressure in adulthood.

4 Change to unrefined, golden granulated sugar instead of white sugar. Reduce sugar in tea, cakes and puddings by around a quarter – use honey or molasses in cooking as an alternative.

Why? Most children in the West today consume far more sugar than is good for them and many consume harmful quantities that can have long term effects on their health.

5 Go organic. Opinion varies on the benefit of organic fruit and vegetables and non-organic is fine if given a good wash before cooking or eating to help remove any traces of pesticides. Meat and dairy products, however, should preferably be organic.

Why? Farm animals are conventionally given artificial hormones to increase milk production or stimulate growth and these can be present in the food they produce.

6 Limit products that have artificial sweetener. Many products that claim to have 'no added sugar' or to be 'low calorie' have just substituted the sugar with sweetener.

Why? Sugar is a natural food that is safe within reasonable limits. Whilst consuming sweeteners or food containing them is acceptable for short term weight loss, the prolonged use of sweeteners has been linked to serious health problems.

7 Cut out hydrogenated margarine and use butter or unhydrogenated margarine (eg Flora) instead. Hydrogenated means that hydrogen has been added to make the spread solid at room temperature.

Why? Research has indicated that these fats may be more dangerous than saturated animal fat. Hydrogenates are high in calories, can affect brain functions such as learning, memory and mood and can also adversely affect the heart.

8 Use only olive oil for frying and cooking, not sunflower, vegetable or any other oil except as a dressing or flavouring.

Why? When some oils are heated they produce free radicals that can damage cells and lead to diseases. Olive oil can withstand high temperatures without the production of free radicals.

9 Switch to free range eggs.

Why? Hens that are allowed to roam freely and scratch for food naturally tend to produce eggs that are healthier than those from hens kept in cages or confined spaces. Some free range eggs also contain omega 3 fatty acids, which may be difficult for children to obtain from their everyday diet.

10 Limit chocolate consumption and try to give organic chocolate wherever possible. Green & Black's organic chocolate is delicious and comes in small bars that are just right for children.

Why? Some chocolate has been found to contain high levels of a dangerous pesticide called lindane, which is linked to impaired immunity and cancer. Although now banned in the EU, lindane is still used in most of the countries that supply the cocoa crop for chocolate. Most chocolate contains high levels of sugar, fat and naturally occurring stimulants that can account for the hyperactivity seen in some children after eating chocolate products.

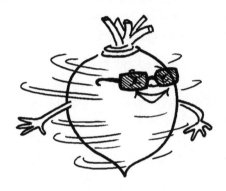

Part **2**

Putting it all
into practice

Being prepared for every occasion can help to ensure that your child eats well throughout the day. This section has ideas to cover most occasions with some recipes included.

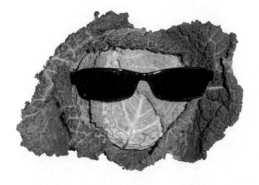

5

Breakfast

This is one of the trickiest times to get down any fruit or vegetables. This is also one of the times when children are most likely to be feeling conservative. If necessary start by eating the following yourself, and ask them to try a bit before having their usual breakfast. Then gradually ask them to try some more in the following weeks.

Here are some easy alternative breakfasts to give your children a healthy start to the day.

• Cereal or toast is so much the norm that changing habits can take time. Make the toast wholemeal if possible and choose cereal that is low in sugar and fat.

• Porridge with whole milk, no sugar and a teaspoon of high-fruit jam (see snacks) is ideal.

• Weekdays, try offering fruit instead of, or with, the usual breakfast cereal. A bowl of tinned fruit in natural juice is a good alternative, followed by some toast to fill up.

• Bananas or strawberries are great with cereal, or chopped into bite size pieces with a warm croissant.

• High fruit jam on toast with tea or fruit juice and a banana makes a good start to the day too.

- Home made flapjacks are healthier than most cereal bars and keep for ages (see puddings and sweet treats).

- On summer mornings try offering yogurt with small pieces of fresh fruit mixed in or a fruit smoothie instead of juice.

- At weekends, grilled tomatoes and mushrooms can be added to poached, boiled or scrambled egg and toast.

Bubble and squeak

Try bubble and squeak occasionally for a treat, or regularly if this is the only way your child will eat leafy green vegetables. Traditionally a way of using leftovers, this dish has recently become very popular again.

A knob of butter
2 or 3 cold boiled potatoes
Some boiled cabbage and/or other cooked vegetables
$1/_2$ onion
1 egg (optional)
A few fresh or dried herbs (optional)

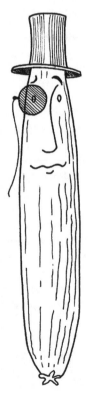

- Heat the butter in a frying pan and gently fry the onion over a low heat until soft.

- Add the vegetables and stir for another couple of minutes.

- Mash the potato well (no lumps) and add to the pan, mixing well with the vegetables.

- Add the egg and herbs at this stage if required.

- Press down the mixture to form a pancake and cook both sides until brown (approx 5 minutes each side).

6

Snacks

If kids come in from school or play and are starving, they want something to eat now, now, NOW! They will not wait while you chop, blend, cook or otherwise prepare anything – they will probably just head for the biscuits or crisps. If you can, it is a good idea to have a menu of food they are allowed to eat anytime as a snack or while waiting for a meal. If you can have emergency snacks on standby, even better. The ideal snack has minimum sugar or salt, will not be gone in one gulp and preferably contains some fruit or vegetable. Serve with fruit juice or high juice squash. Here are some ideas that you can experiment with. Combine two or three if your child is extra hungry.

- A milkshake or smoothie (see drinks)

- A small roll or one sandwich with some salad sticks (carrot, cucumber, celery and perhaps some cherry tomatoes and chopped apple)

- A couple of home made cakes or muffins (with hidden fruit), already prepared

- A small packet or handful of raisins

- A banana

- Plain biscuits (eg rich tea or digestives)

- Dip made of yogurt, finely chopped cucumber and a teaspoon of mint sauce, with wholemeal pitta bread or a few chicken breast pieces to dip in it

- A yoghurt (not the high sugar fromage frais) with some small fruit to dip, fresh fruit pieces or mashed banana added

- A couple of crackers with cheese and salad sticks

- A bowl of strawberries or raspberries

- One or two satsumas

- Brown bread and butter topped with high fruit, no added sugar jam such as Thursday Cottage or St Dalfour (available from health food shops and large supermarkets)

- A chopped apple

- A bunch of grapes

- A fruit juice ice lolly (just freeze fruit juice into lolly moulds)

- A cereal bar (most parents can find one that their child likes and is not too sweet)

- Mashed banana sandwich with an optional drizzle of honey

- Cheese on toast (preferably brown bread and with salad, of course)

- A bowl of popcorn (not the really sweet toffee one you buy in a bag but the make-it-yourself on the hob or in the microwave variety)

- A small bowl of cereal (without added sugar)

- Cream cheese or dip with salad sticks & cherry tomatoes

- French bread slice with butter and salad

- A handful of plain nuts (not salted or roasted)

- Pure fruit bars (concentrated fruit with no added sugar is best eg Humzingers, or School Bars available from supermarkets)

- A kiwi fruit, cut in half to eat with a spoon

- A small jacket potato or sweet potato with butter (quick to make in the microwave)

- A bowl of tinned fruit (in natural juice, not syrup)

- Bread sticks with butter or cheese spread and (you guessed it) salad sticks

- Pretzels (lower in salt and fat than most crisps)

- Houmous with wholemeal pitta bread

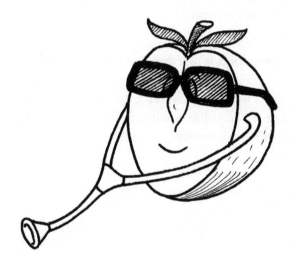

7

Main meals for the family

It is worth saying again how important it is for children to eat together with adults, even once a week, in order to learn to eat grown-up food. However, in practice it can be so difficult to prepare a meal that everyone likes.

Presenting a variety of food to choose from so that children can help themselves means that they can take just as much as they are prepared to eat, leave what they don't and there is less waste. Invest in a few large bowls with lids to keep food hot at the table, and a couple of washable or wipe clean tablecloths. Good family meals have plenty of variety.

Chilli con carne with corn bread

A mild chilli is a hit with most children and is a good winter warmer. Corn bread is easy to make and the children can help with this.

2 tablespoons olive oil
1 large onion, finely chopped
2 cloves garlic, crushed
Approx 1lb/450g mince (lean beef, lamb, chicken or quorn)
Large can tomatoes, blended

1 tablespoon concentrated tomato purée
1 teaspoon chilli powder
2 heaped teaspoons fresh or dried mixed herbs
1 can of red kidney beans, drained

- Fry the onion and garlic in the olive oil until soft.

- Add the mince and cook for approx 5-10 minutes.

- Add tomatoes, purée, herbs and chilli powder.

- Cover the pan and bring to the boil. Add a little boiling water at this stage if the mixture is looking stodgy or sticking to the bottom of the pan.

- Reduce the heat to low and cook for approx 30 minutes.

- Add the kidney beans, cover the pan and simmer on a low heat for another 20 minutes.

Serve with:
- Tacos or wraps
- Salad made with mild onion, tomato, cucumber and grated carrot
- Corn chips
- Guacamole (avocado) dip
- Grated cheese
- Rice (see tips for cooking rice below under curry)

Corn bread

4 tablespoons olive oil
1 small can sweetcorn
6 tablespoons cornmeal
$1/2$ teaspoon low sodium salt
2-3 teaspoons baking powder
2 eggs
A little butter and plain flour

$^1/_4$pt/150ml single cream
$^1/_2$ finely chopped onion (optional)
8oz/225g grated cheese

• Beat the eggs and oil together.

• Add the sweetcorn, cream and salt – mix well.

• Mix in the cornmeal and baking powder.

• Add most of the cheese with onions if using and give a good stir.

• Grease a baking tin with butter and add enough flour to stop the mixture sticking.

• Add the mixture, sprinkle the last of the cheese on top and cook in a low-medium oven (180/350/gas 4) for about 45 minutes.

• Turn out when slightly cooled and cut into slices – serve warm.

Summer supper

This is a great family meal and a good mix of healthy things to eat.

First, make sure that everyone has washed their hands as everything will be well handled before eating.

You don't have to use everything on the list, just use what you have. Arrange everything attractively on large plates or trays on the table. Talk, play and trust that adequate amounts of healthy things actually make it into the tummies of your children. They will love to make pictures and faces on their plates with the food they have selected before eating the wheels/hair/chimney of their masterpiece.

French stick, cut into small slices & lightly buttered
Shredded lettuce
The smallest cherry tomatoes
Strips of red, yellow and orange pepper

Seedless grapes
Some thin carrot sticks
A whole cucumber cut into generous chunks
Sliced avocado
A few hard boiled eggs, peeled and cut in half
Shelled nuts (not for very young children)
Raisins
Some raw onion rings
A generous pile of mustard and cress
A bowl of grated cheese and/or some sticks of cheese
Slices of cold meat – ham, salami, liver sausage, chicken
Chicken drumsticks, hot or cold
A plate of potato or sweet potato wedges (recipe below)
A variety of dips
Mayonnaise
Ketchup

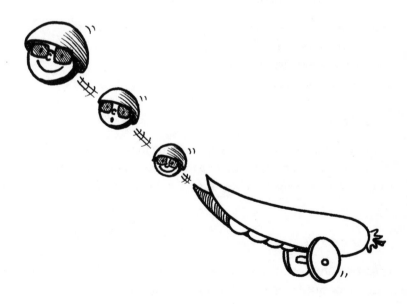

Fajitas

Easy to prepare, either selecting your own ingredients or using pre-packed kits they make a satisfying weekend dinner.

Use lots of sliced onions, well cooked until soft (include slices of garlic). Thinly slice meat or chicken, and stir-fry with vegetables (eg peppers, carrots) and sauce from a jar or packet.

Serve with:
• Soft flour tortillas
• Grated cheese
• Potato wedges (see below)
• Sour cream
• Shredded lettuce
• Salsa

Mild salsa

You can use ready made salsa or try this recipe:

1 large can tomatoes, drained and mashed or blended
1 large mild onion, finely chopped or blended
2 fresh, ripe tomatoes, finely diced
$\frac{1}{2}$ teaspoon low sodium salt
1 pinch black pepper
1 dash Tabasco or teaspoon of sweet chilli sauce (optional)

Combine ingredients in a saucepan, bring to the boil and boil rapidly for 1-2 minutes, then remove from heat. Cool and keep in the fridge for up to 4 weeks. This sauce also freezes well.

Egg fried rice

1 cup long grain or basmati rice – washed and drained (an average teacup or small mug is enough for a family of 3-4).

2 cups of water
1 clove garlic
3 tablespoons olive oil
3 eggs
1 bunch spring onions, very finely chopped
1 bunch coriander, finely chopped and divided into 3 portions
$^1/_2$ cup frozen petits pois
2 tablespoons dark soy sauce
1 heaped teaspoon low sodium salt
A little white or black pepper

• Boil the water in a large pan and add the rice but switch off heat once the water is absorbed. Wait for 2 minutes then turn the rice out on to a large plate to stop it cooking further or sticking.

• Mix the eggs and season with a little salt and pepper.

• Add $^1/_3$ of the spring onions and half the coriander.

• Heat some of the oil and fry the egg mixture, making a thin omelette. When cooked and slightly brown underneath, turn the omelette out on to a plate, roll it up and shred it as finely as possible.

• In a large wok, fry the garlic, remaining spring onions, petits pois and $^2/_3$ of the coriander in the rest of the oil, stir-frying for 1 minute.

• Add the rice, shredded egg and soy sauce and stir-fry for a further 5 minutes. Garnish with the remaining coriander and serve immediately.

This rice is tasty enough to be served on its own but can be eaten with any Chinese dish or stir-fry. If preparing a home cooked stir-fry include beansprouts and plenty of fresh, shredded vegetables. Alternatively, serve with prepared dishes from the supermarket or takeaway if you are short of time.

Chicken Curry

1 onion and 1 clove garlic, finely chopped or blended
2 chicken breasts, chopped into small pieces
$^1/_2$ finely shredded or blended red pepper
1 heaped tablespoon fresh or dried coriander
A generous squeeze tomato purée
3 dessert spoons plain yogurt
Curry powder, paste or sauce according to taste

- Fry the onions, pepper and garlic.

- Add the chicken and fry until lightly brown.

- Add the curry flavouring, tomato purée, half the coriander and a little boiling water if necessary – bring to the boil and cook for 5-10 minutes, stirring regularly.

- Turn the heat to low, add the yogurt and stir well.

- Garnish with the remaining coriander.

Serve with:
- Sliced tomatoes, cucumber and onion
- Raita (plain yogurt with chopped or grated cucumber mixed in)
- Naan bread, pitta bread or chapattis
- Rice with peas

Tips for cooking rice

Rice is easy to cook, a great standby and makes a change from potatoes. The basic rules for cooking rice are:

- Soak it first for at least 10 minutes, stir and drain off the starchy water (this prevents the rice from being too sticky).

- Use one cup of rice to two cups of water.

- Use a saucepan with a well fitting lid.

- Boil the water first then add the rice – if you put the rice in the pan first it can stick to the pan and burn.

- Add a little salt.

- Add frozen peas and/or sweetcorn after the water has boiled.

- When most of the water has been absorbed, switch off the heat but leave the lid on for 10 minutes – the rice will continue cooking but not overcook.

- Garnish with finely chopped coriander.

- Serve immediately if possible and always eat within 24 hours of cooking. Reheat thoroughly as cold rice is notorious for harbouring bugs and causing tummy aches.

If you want to introduce brown rice, which has more fibre, into your child's diet, first try making the usual white rice with half a teaspoon of turmeric, added just after the rice has been added to the water. After a while, yellow rice will seem normal and you can start replacing one tenth of the white rice with brown rice (check the cooking times as the brown rice may need to go in first) – it will all be yellow and look the same. Gradually increase the proportion of brown rice and decrease the white.

Risotto

An all-in-one dish that you can add almost anything to, risotto is satisfying and although time consuming to make it is worth it for a meal that you can cook in one pan. Use short grain rice – special risotto rice is available in supermarkets.

1 medium onion
vegetables according to preference and availability
$^1/_2$ tablespoon olive oil
8-10oz/250-300g rice approx

$^1/_2$pt-1pt/300-500ml stock
optional chopped, cooked meat or fish
salt and pepper to season
freshly chopped herbs of your choice
2-3oz/75g parmesan cheese
1oz/30g butter

- First fry one onion and any other uncooked vegetable you wish in some butter or olive oil until it is soft. You could fry carrot, pumpkin, mushrooms, tomatoes, garlic etc with the onion.

- Add the rice, about 2oz per child and a little more for each adult, then stir-fry with the vegetables for about 2 minutes.

- Make some hot stock, around 2 cups for every one cup of rice, and add a little at a time, starting with a cupful, and stir into the mixture until absorbed.

- Meat, chicken, fish or soft vegetables, such as peas, can be added at this stage.

- Add more stock gradually, stirring frequently to prevent the rice from sticking – you do need to stand over it and may get an aching arm from the continuous stirring required.

Once all the stock is absorbed season with salt, pepper and freshly chopped herbs. Add a little parmesan cheese and some butter, stir in and serve immediately.

Pasta

A basic tomato sauce is quick to make and can be served with any shaped pasta, dried or fresh and cooked in lightly salted water until soft. The recipe can be varied to include fresh tomatoes, tomato purée, any fresh herbs and some finely chopped and well disguised vegetables. Use this for the basic sauce and add whatever additional healthy ingredients you have:

1 large onion, peeled and chopped
2-3 cloves crushed garlic
2 tablespoons olive oil
2 cans chopped plum tomatoes
2 handfuls chopped basil leaves

- Heat the oil and fry the chopped onion with the garlic until soft.

- Add the tomatoes to the saucepan and heat through until bubbling.

- Add the basil, stir then cover the pan.

- Simmer on a low heat for about 30-45 minutes, stirring occasionally.

- Meanwhile, cook and drain the pasta.

- Pour over the sauce and top with a little parmesan or grated cheese.

Serve with:
- Garlic bread
- Mixed salad

Pizza

Whether you make your own base or use ready made ones, you can still get plenty of healthy things into the topping. The basic topping can be made using the same ingredients as the pasta sauce (above) but using less liquid and reducing if necessary – do this by just boiling rapidly until it becomes thicker.

8oz/225g self raising flour (substitute half wholemeal flour for extra fibre)
4 tablespoons of olive oil
1 heaped dessert spoon dried mixed herbs
$1/2$ teaspoon low sodium salt
A little water

- Sift the flour and salt into a bowl. Add the herbs and mix.

- Make a well in the centre of the mixture and pour in half the olive oil and a little water. Mix into a soft dough gradually adding more water if required.

- Roll out on a floured surface until you have a circle to fit your largest frying pan – non-stick with shallow or sloping sides is best.

- Add 1 tablespoon of olive oil to the pan and heat.

- Place the dough in the pan and cook for about 4 minutes over a low heat.

- When the underside is light brown, turn it out onto a plate, add the remaining oil to the pan and cook the other side of the base.

- When almost ready, add the basic topping sauce, a variety of vegetables* and some grated or thinly sliced cheese. Top with a drizzle of olive oil.

- Place the frying pan under a medium grill for a few minutes until the topping is hot and the cheese bubbles – serve immediately with garlic bread and a mixed salad.

*Optional toppings:
- Sweetcorn kernels, fresh or from a can
- Sliced olives
- Sliced mushrooms
- Shredded peppers – various colours
- Onion rings or slices
- A variety of fresh herbs – fresh basil tastes great on pizza
- Sliced tomatoes

Serve with:
- Garlic bread
- Mixed salad

Potato Wedges

Wedges are healthier than chips and keeping the skin on means extra fibre. They are versatile and can be served with many savoury dishes.

1-2 medium potatoes per person
Olive oil
Salt
1 tablespoon dried mixed herbs

- Scrub 1 or 2 medium potatoes per person and cut in half. Place each half on a chopping board with the flat side facing down. Slice each half into three lengthways with the cuts all meeting in the middle of the base.

- When all the wedges have been cut, put them into a bowl of water to soak for at least 30 minutes then drain them and pat dry.

- Put a generous slug of olive oil in a bowl, add a rounded table-spoon of dried mixed herbs and a level teaspoon of salt.

- Toss the potato wedges in the oil mixture until they are completely coated – add more olive oil if you need to.

- Put the wedges into a baking tray with the skin side down and cook in the oven 200/400/gas 6 for around 25 minutes or until brown and soft in the middle.

Wedges can also be made with sweet potato, which is richer in nutrients and fibre.

8

Meals for children

There will always be occasions when only children need to be fed, and it is tempting to do the quickest thing possible.

Fish fingers and chips are OK, but grill rather than fry them and serve with peas, sweetcorn and carrots rather than tinned spaghetti. Make jacket potatoes or mash, and cook oven chips rather than fried. Serving baked beans rather than spaghetti is preferable as beans do at least have some fibre.

Beans on toast made with wholemeal bread is a substantial snack for a small child. Try the healthy option baked beans as they have less sugar and salt (but check the label as some contain sweeteners), then add some tomato purée before heating to improve the taste if necessary.

Make and freeze **mini sized pizzas**.

Cook **dried pasta shapes** with your own tomato sauce or one from a jar with any extra vegetables that you can slip in.

Sausage and bean casserole

This has lots of fibre and can be made quickly with minimum effort.

1 small onion
Olive oil
1 tablespoon tomato purée
$1/_4$ cup water
1 large tin of baked beans with pork or vegetarian sausages
1 small tin sweetcorn (preferably without added salt and sugar)
Grated cheese (optional)

- Chop the onion and fry in olive oil for about 5 minutes.

- Stir in the tomato purée and water.

- After another 5 minutes add the tin of baked beans with sausages (Heinz do one called 'Healthy Balance' with vegetable sausages and lower levels of salt and sugar) and the tin of sweetcorn.

- Warm through thoroughly and serve with jacket potato or mash and top with grated cheese.

- Alternatively, put the hot bean mixture into a dish, sprinkle with cheese and place in a medium oven for about 15 minutes.

- Serves two children.

Soup

With a roll or crusty bread, soup is a substantial snack or light meal for children. Tinned soups can be high in salt and sugar though. Fresh soup is widely available in supermarkets and can have a better flavour. Try blending for a few seconds if there are lumps that your child might not like. Home made soup is obviously preferable, but can be time consuming to make. Most do freeze well, however.

Pumpkin soup

1 medium onion, peeled and chopped
2 garlic cloves, crushed
Olive oil
1 small pumpkin or large butternut squash
1 large carrot
1 bay leaf
1pt/500ml stock
1 level teaspoon cumin powder (optional)
$1/4$pt/150ml cream (optional)
Croutons, grated cheese or chopped herbs to garnish

- Fry the onion in a large saucepan with olive oil and crushed garlic cloves until soft.

- Peel and chop the pumpkin or butternut squash and the carrot.

- Add them to the onion with a bay leaf and half a pint of stock.

- A level teaspoon of cumin powder added at this stage gives a lovely warming flavour.

- When the soup starts to bubble, cover and cook on a low heat for about 30-45 minutes, stirring once or twice to make sure it doesn't stick to the bottom of the pan.

- Turn off the heat and leave to cool for about 10 minutes, then blend or mash all of the liquid until smooth.

- Stir in the cream and reheat well.

- Serve immediately garnished with croutons, grated cheese or chopped fresh herbs.

Tomato and basil soup

1 large tin chopped plum tomatoes
1 onion, peeled and chopped
Olive oil
2 heaped tablespoons chopped fresh basil
1 cup of water
$1/2$ teaspoon sugar
$1/4$pt/150ml cream (optional)
Seasoning

- Drain the tin of tomatoes (keep the juice).

- Fry the chopped onion in olive oil until soft.

- Add the tomatoes and basil, some salt and pepper, and cook for 1 minute.

- Add the tomato juice, water and sugar. Stir well.

- Simmer for 10 minutes, cool slightly then mash or blend the liquid.

- Reheat uncovered until the soup thickens, then add the cream and warm through before serving.

Croutons

Soups are more tempting for reluctant children, and a little more filling, if you add croutons. These can be bought in packets but tend to be quite salty. Alternatively, you can make croutons easily at home and they keep very well in the freezer.

2 tablespoons dried herbs
5 tablespoons olive oil
pinch salt
6 slices thick sliced, slightly stale bread

- Turn the oven on to hot.

- Stir the dried herbs into the olive oil with a pinch of salt.

- Remove the crusts from the bread and cut into cubes.

- Toss the bread cubes in the oil mixture then spread the cubes on a lined or greased baking tray.

- Bake for around 15-20 minutes, turning over once so that they cook evenly.

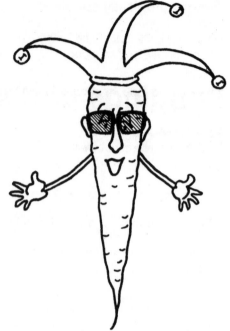

- Add to soups and salads – they keep for three weeks in the fridge or much longer in the freezer.

Try making your own bread to go with soup. You can add sundried tomatoes, dried fruit (apricot bread goes well with pumpkin soup) or fresh chopped herbs, or hide other dried or preserved fruit and vegetables. Served hot your kids will find it hard to resist.

9

Puddings and sweet treats

Pancakes are a quick and filling dessert. Serve with stewed fruit filling or grate an apple or pear into the pancake mix before cooking. Squeeze fresh lemon juice over the top and garnish with lemon or orange slices.

Banana custard is an old favourite that is still popular, especially if introduced to children at a young age – use plenty of banana chopped into small pieces and if making your own custard try adding less sugar.

Stewed fruit has gone out of fashion in recent years but is a great way to maintain fruit levels in winter. Use eating apples instead of the cooking variety and you need hardly add any sugar at all. Rhubarb is also high in fibre. Serve stewed fruit with a milk pudding or custard.

Apple pie is often high in sugar and ready made ones usually contain hydrogenated fat in the pastry. If you make your own pastry, use unhydrogenated margarine, cover the top only with pastry, don't have a base, and use more fruit and less sugar than your recipe suggests. Serve with a little cream or organic ice cream.

Fruit sorbets

Sorbets can be made from almost any fruit and are a low fat, low sugar but delicious and light dessert. Although easier with an ice cream maker, just stirring a few times during freezing produces the same result. Experiment with exotic fruit such as mango and pineapple and use up fruit that is in season.

Strawberry sorbet

1 punnet ripe strawberries
2 tablespoons honey
1 small pot natural yoghurt
1 tablespoon lemon juice

- Purée the strawberries in a food processor or blender.

- Add the honey, lemon and yogurt – stir well.

- Add to the ice cream maker or put into a solid tub in the freezer, taking out occasionally to stir.

As a treat, make **banana splits** with ripe bananas, a scoop of organic ice cream, a little honey, syrup or fruit purée drizzled over and some small strawberries or raspberries on top.

Chocolate dipped fruit

This is a great treat for parties and a lovely summer dessert for children. They will also enjoy helping you to make it.

- Take around 6oz/175g of organic chocolate and a selection of washed and dried soft fruit – strawberries, cherries, satsuma segments, grapes, pineapple chunks.

- Melt the chocolate in a small bowl, either over a pan of hot water or in the microwave.

- Spear each piece of fruit with a cocktail stick and dip it in the chocolate, covering at least half of the fruit.

- Leave the covered fruit pieces to set on waxed paper.

- Serve when completely set, arranged on a tray or plate. For special occasions and parties, place each fruit piece in a small paper sweet case.

Flapjacks

These make a filling snack and are much healthier than chocolate and most cereal bars. Try this basic recipe:

4oz/100g softened butter or unhydrogenated margarine
3oz/75g golden caster sugar
10oz/275g oats
2 tablespoons honey
Some chopped dried apricots
A handful of raisins

- Combine all the ingredients in a bowl. Add a mashed banana as an optional extra if the flapjacks will be eaten the same day.

- Put the mixture into a greased baking tray, press down hard then bake on a medium heat 180°/350°/gas 4 for approx 25 minutes.

- Cool slightly, cut into squares and serve or keep in an airtight container for up to a week.

Cakes and muffins

Cakes and muffins are a great way to hide fruit. Grate, chop or cook and mash the fruit before adding to your normal cake mixture. By including fruit in your recipes you can reduce the sugar by about one quarter. Many types of dried or fresh fruit can be used – prunes are particularly good (and easy to hide) in chocolate cake. Carrots also have a sweet flavour and can add nutrition and fibre to cakes.

Banana and apricot loaf

This is a favourite and great for tea time and picnics, but best straight from the oven, sliced into chunks, spread with butter and topped with a little jam or honey. (You can halve the baking time by cooking individual cakes in a greased muffin tin.)

8oz/225g self raising flour
4oz/100g non-hydrogenated margarine
3oz/75g golden granulated or soft brown sugar
2 large eggs
$1/2$ teaspoon baking powder
$1/4$ teaspoon ground cinnamon or nutmeg
3 very ripe bananas, peeled and mashed
About 6oz/175g ready-to-eat dried apricots, chopped into small pieces

- Heat the oven to 180°/350°/gas 4.

- Beat the sugar, margarine and eggs together, then add the flour, baking powder and spices and combine well.

- Stir in the mashed banana and chopped apricots and bake in a greased loaf tin for about $1^1/4$ hours.

- Cool slightly before turning out.

Chocolate rice crispy cakes

These are always a hit with children and great for parties or picnics. Make them healthier by using organic chocolate and adding a handful of dried, stoned prunes.

4oz/100g organic milk chocolate
1lb/500g crisped rice cereal

handful dried, stoned prunes or a small tin of prunes
zest of 1 medium orange

- Blend the prunes well or chop into very small pieces.

- Melt the chocolate and add the prunes when the chocolate is still warm. Add the orange zest for extra flavour.

- Stir in the cereal.

- Set in small cake cases or in a tray for cutting into kiddie sized chunks.

Real fruit **ice lollies** are cooling and hydrating in the summer and also contain vitamin C. Simply pour fresh juice into lolly moulds and freeze for at least three hours. Experiment with different juices and add yogurt, milk, honey or blended fresh fruit for variety of flavours – children love helping with this.

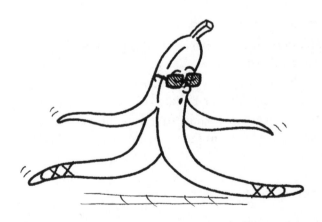

Drinks

Fruit juice can be freshly squeezed, which is best, but long life juice is better than fizzy drinks or squash. Juicers make it easy to extract juice from a wide range of fruit – and vegetables too. Children can help to choose which fruit to juice and put the fruit pieces into the juicer.

Watch out for sweetened drinks, usually in cartons, labelled 'juice drink'. These contain only a small percentage of juice with added sugar and water.

Squash often contains high levels of sugar. The high juice varieties are better. Add some pure juice of the same colour to the squash before diluting, roughly 1 part squash, 2 parts juice and five parts filtered water. In summer, replace the water with sparkling mineral water, add ice cubes made from pure juice and slices of orange and lemon. Keep a jug in the fridge for all day cool drinks.

Real lemonade

This may be high in sugar but has no artificial sweeteners or preservatives. Make it fresh and keep it cool for the best taste:

2pts/1l of filtered water

4oz/100g golden granulated or caster sugar
5 lemons

- Put water and sugar into a jug and mix well until all the sugar is dissolved – you may need to warm the water slightly.

- Squeeze the juice from 4 of the lemons and add to the water and sugar.

- Wash and slice the remaining lemon and add the slices to the jug.

- Chill for at least 1 hour before serving.

Fresh lemonade, kept cold in a flask, is also great for picnics and lunchboxes.

Smoothies

There is a variety of smoothie makers on the market to make smoothie creation easier. You don't actually need a smoothie maker, however, to make smoothies – an ordinary blender can work quite well. Use any soft, ripe fruit in any combination that your children like. Children will enjoy experimenting with you and are usually happy to consume the results, especially if they have a chance to invent their own recipes. Here are a few ideas for smoothie ingredients – just blend well and serve immediately or chill and consume within 24 hours.

Mango smoothie

1 large or 2 small very ripe mangoes, peeled, chopped and chilled
1 ripe banana, peeled and chilled
2 fl oz/55ml milk
3 scoops vanilla or banana ice cream
1-2 teaspoons honey

Pineapple smoothie

1 small tin pineapple slices or chunks
2fl oz/55ml pineapple juice
I ripe banana, peeled and chilled
1 small carton natural yogurt

Strawberry smoothie

12-15 strawberries, washed and with stalks removed
2 ripe bananas, peeled, chopped and frozen overnight
$^{1}/_{2}$pt/300ml milk or $^{1}/_{4}$pt/150ml apple juice

Milkshakes are a satisfying drink, and the froth can also hide a multitude of things – think vitamin drops, probiotics, omega oils and even prescription medicines...

There is no need to use commercial milkshake mixes that contain lots of sugar – add any soft fruit, fresh or canned, to provide the sweetness. You can sieve out any pips to make it smoother and add a scoop of ice cream or a little honey to improve the taste.

Here are a couple of easy milkshakes:

Banana milkshake

1 Banana
$^{1}/_{2}$pt/300ml milk
Small scoop organic vanilla or banana ice cream

- Cut a peeled ripe banana into small chunks and then freeze it for a few hours

- Add to the milk and blend well

- Add the ice cream and blend in too or just float on top

Peach milkshake

1 small can peaches in natural juice
1 small pot plain yogurt
$^1/_2$pt/300ml milk
1 level teaspoon sugar (optional)

• Blend the peaches in a blender.

• Add the milk, sugar and yoghurt and blend until frothy.

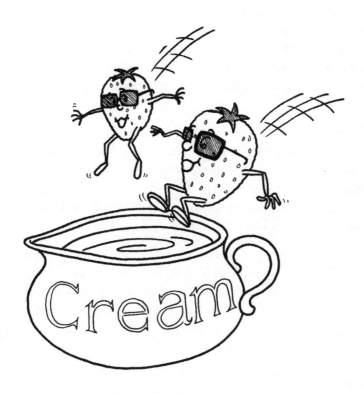

Packed lunches

The advantage of giving your children a packed lunch for school is that they have little choice but to eat what you provide – or go hungry. The disadvantage is that they will often choose what they want to eat and leave the rest, and sometimes will go hungry rather than try something new or eat something they are not keen on.

You can go some way to avoiding this by making up the lunchbox after consulting your children and asking them to help with the choosing and packing. Get them to try new things in advance by having a tasting session. Make mini sandwiches, snacks and cakes then ask them to select the ones they like best and tell you the ones they really don't want to eat.

The main objective for children when eating lunch at school is to finish it as quickly as possible so they can get outside to play. Don't overfill lunchboxes as this might be daunting and lead to lots of wasted food. Here are a few other ideas to help ensure that your child consumes at least something healthy at school and comes home with an empty lunchbox.

Sandwiches

Make sandwiches with wholemeal or half-and-half bread (see parties below). Cut into quarters or different shapes with pastry or biscuit cutters for younger children. If your children don't like crusts *cut them off*. There is no point in trying to force children to eat crusts.

As a change from bread you can use **bagels, tortilla wraps** or **pitta bread pockets** – all are widely available and can be purchased in mini sizes for smaller appetites. Or you could put a filling inside rice cakes – especially useful if you have a child with a wheat allergy.

Limit fillings that are high in fat and salt, such as ham or mayonnaise. Healthier basic fillings include:

• Free-range boiled *eggs* mashed with a little low sodium salt and mixed together with olive oil instead of mayonnaise.

• Home cooked *meat or poultry*, well cooked and thoroughly cooled, is healthier and lower in salt than pre-packed sliced meat.

• *Tuna* – mash it with a little olive oil plus a teaspoon of mayonnaise and add a tablespoon of cooked sweetcorn.

• *Cheese* can be grated and used sparingly – organic is preferable. *Cream cheese* is also tasty and not much is needed.

• *Peanut butter* may be an acquired taste but many kids love it once they try it.

• *Marmite* is a good source of B vitamins but spread thinly as it is very salty.

• *Humous* is a savoury Greek dip and filling that many children enjoy if they can be persuaded to taste it – now available in most supermarkets.

Always try to add a little *salad*, preferably grated or shredded to prevent children taking out slices and larger chunks:

• *Coleslaw* is a great way to include ready prepared salad in sandwiches (you can also just give them a pot of it and a spoon to eat it with).

- *Cress* is easy to chew and has a mild flavour – if children grow this themselves they will be much more likely to eat it.

- Slice *cucumber* thinly.

- Shred *lettuce* finely.

- Include the smallest cherry *tomatoes* that will be sweet and easy to chew.

- For the really fussy ones, mix red cheese such as Leicester together with finely grated *carrot* – the filling will then all look the same.

Other lunchbox foods

- *Mini pizzas* are popular with most children and a tasty alternative to bread. Make a batch and freeze in advance for convenience and speed.

- Older children will feel really grown-up if they are given a *mixed salad* in a small container with a well fitting lid. A simple dressing of extra virgin olive oil, a little low sodium salt and some dried or finely chopped herbs adds flavour. Add croutons, home made or shop bought, to make it more filling.

- Your child may eat sticks of *carrot, cucumber, pepper* or *celery* if you give them something to dip it in. You can use cream cheese, or make a dip from fromage frais and ketchup with a few herbs; or yogurt, cucumber and mint sauce (see 'snacks'). If your child helps make the dip, they're more likely to eat it.

- Free range *hard-boiled eggs*, already peeled and cut in half, can be eaten on their own, in a salad or with a dip.

- Sliced cold *chicken or meats* and cold *mini sausages* can be given as finger food rather than sandwich fillings.

Savoury nibbles

These help to fill your child up.

- *Crisps* are often high in salt and fat, but including them in lunchboxes once or twice a week is OK – try organic or low salt varieties.

- As an alternative, *pretzels* are lower in fat.

- *Tortilla chips* that are plain or just lightly salted can be given with a small pot of salsa for dipping.

- Salty *popcorn* has the added advantage of counting as a vegetable and is high in fibre.

- *Nuts and seeds* make a healthy snack if your child is not allergic, but check with the school as some don't allow nuts.

Fruit

Always try to include one portion of fruit in a lunchbox. If it is fresh, make sure your child can open it easily. Oranges can take ages to peel and bananas can be difficult to break so start them off by making a small cut in the skin. Fruit can also be ready peeled and prepared and then wrapped in clingfilm. Pack small fresh fruit into little bags, or small containers if they are likely to squash easily.

- *Tinned fruit* in natural juice makes a nice change – put into a small container with a good lid (and don't forget to add a spoon).

- *Jelly* with added fruit in small containers can be made in advance. Fruit pots and jelly with added fruit by Dole, Del Monte and Fruitini can be purchased in most supermarkets.

- Chopped fresh fruit can also be added to *yogurt* or used to dip into yoghurt or fromage frais.

- A variety of *dried fruit* can be given in lunchboxes – think beyond raisins and try your child with apricots, prunes and even banana. There are also snacks made from pure fruit with no added sugar – School Bars and Humzingers are naturally sweet and healthy.

- *Fruit purée* makes a delicious change from yogurt. Clearspring produce four flavours of apple purée that is organic and without additives or added sugar – can be purchased from health food shops or online.

Small children may be unable to chew and swallow apple skin, but peeled apple goes brown quite quickly. Avoid this by chopping it into bite size pieces after peeling, and wrapping it in foil.

Keep it cool

It goes without saying that food should be packed as cold as possible, especially in warm weather, to prevent it from harbouring bugs and tasting yukky. Insulated lunchboxes with ice packs or soft ice mats to wrap around food or drinks can help to keep everything chilled until lunchtime during summer.

Make it hot

In winter, however, it can be miserable for children to eat cold food then go out into the cold to play, especially if they are eating together with others who have hot lunch. Flasks are not just for tea and come in a variety of sizes and widths for drinks or food.

- A small flask of *tea* or *hot, milky drink* can be comforting on a cold day. Squash can also be made with hot water and kept warm until lunchtime. Warm the flask with boiling water first then tip it out and immediately add the piping hot drink, filling the flask to the top. Put the lid on straight away and the drink will still be satisfyingly hot at lunchtime.

- *Soup* is warming and satisfying, so is warmed vegetable baby food, on its own or added to tomato soup, handy for kids who don't like lumpy soup.

- Flasks can also be used to keep *pasta* or even *roast vegetables* hot. Don't forget to pack a small bowl and a spoon.

Sweet treats

You can include one sweet treat a day.

- *Cakes* or muffins with added fruit (see puddings and sweet treats) can be made in large quantities and frozen – just take one or two out of the freezer in the morning as required.

- *Sesame snaps* are quite high in sugar but are dairy and wheat free – great for children with these allergies.

- *Cereal bars* can also be high in sugar, and try to avoid ones with hydrogenated fats. Organic varieties include Doves Farm cereal bars (available from Waitrose, Tesco and health food shops) which come in 'cornflake and fruit' or 'rice pop and chocolate' flavours.

- *Flapjacks* are easy to make, keep for longer than cakes and have more fibre. If buying ready made flapjacks, choose ones that do not have hydrogenated fat.

- A square of *chocolate rice crispy cake* (see puddings and sweet treats) is sure to go down well.

- *Yogurts* can be tasty and nutritious but try to buy ones with added fruit that are not too sweet. Alternatively, put some natural yoghurt into a small pot and swirl honey or high fruit jam into it or add chopped fresh fruit. If your child doesn't like lumps and you don't have much time, puréed fruit baby food spooned into a little natural yogurt adds sweetness and nutrition.

- Although it doesn't contain any fruit, a small bar of *organic chocolate* for an extra treat now and again will be welcome – Green & Black's do lovely small bars that are becoming widely available. Delvaux petit organique are small, organic, individually wrapped chocolate squares and good value at £2.99 for 24 (minimum order six). Add one or two once a week for a treat your children will love. Available from the Delvaux web site (see **whiteladderpress.com** for details).

Lunchbox drinks

Ensure that home made drinks are packed in bottles or flasks with well fitting lids (see drinks for ideas). Cartons of pure juice are a practical standby and now that mineral water comes in small sports bottles this has become an acceptably cool lunchbox drink.

Chill cold drinks overnight in the fridge before packing in the morning. During hot weather, try putting the bottle in the freezer for an hour before you pack it to make it really icy.

Smoothies count as a drink and fruit. They can also be quite filling. If you make your own keep them well chilled and use within two days. Healthier ready made smoothies include PJ's and Soma (flavours include fruity roots and jungle juice) – both are available from most major health food shops and web sites. PJ's smoothies are also available at some larger supermarkets. The Juice Company makes Smile Smoothies and SmoothiePack, both in a variety of delicious flavours.

Parties

Children's parties are generally associated with cake, jelly and ice cream, which are high in fat, sugar or both and with almost no nutritional value. Making some adjustments to the food served at parties can increase the nutrition and lower the hyperactivity of children after eating.

Sandwiches that are served at parties can be made with wholemeal bread for increased fibre and nutrition, or with one of the half-and-half varieties (Kingsmill Wholemeal and White, Hovis Best of Both). Alternatively, sandwiches made with one white and one brown slice look interesting and attractive.

You can also cut sandwiches for parties into different shapes. Add some light salad to the fillings too – cress, grated carrot, finely chopped herbs or some thinly sliced cucumber.

Open sandwiches

These look great and this encourages the children to eat them. Your own children will want to help make them too. Use any combinations of the following to top your open sandwiches:

- Slices of cheddar cut into rounds to fit the bread
- Slices of hard boiled egg cut crosswise to give a round rather than oval shape

- Slices of ham cut into rounds
- Cream cheese spread on the bread
- Meat or vegetable paté spread on the bread
- Slices of cucumber
- Slices of tomato
- Half a grape
- Slice of pitted black olive sliced across to give a hole in the middle

Cut the bread into rounds using a cookie cutter and butter each round.

On top of each round place a combination of the ingredients listed below so that each one looks different. You might have a round of cheese with a slice of egg on one, and a round of ham with a slice of tomato on the next, and so on.

You can use a little blob of mayonnaise to get them to stick together.

Crisps can be replaced by snacks that are lower in salt – pretzels or tortilla chips served with healthy dips (see salsa, above, under fajitas in main meals for the family).

Salad Add salad sticks and cherry tomatoes to the plates of sandwiches and also place next to the dips.

Mini pizzas are always popular – use the pizza recipe above or, to save time making bases, use muffins cut in half.

Jellies and trifles It is preferable to use jelly mixture that does not include gelatine, an animal by-product, as a setting agent – there are several other options available in supermarkets. Generally it is better to use a jelly mixture sweetened with sugar, not sweeteners. Add tinned fruit in natural juice to the jelly or trifle bowl before pouring on the jelly. Alternatively, pour hot water over some soft fresh fruit (strawberries, raspberries, grapes etc) before adding the jelly mixture. Make the jelly with a small amount of very hot water to dissolve and top up the rest of the liquid with fruit juice. Decorate jellies and trifles with small pieces of fresh fruit.

Serve **fruit sorbet** (see puddings and sweet treats) as an alternative to ice cream.

Cakes Use a recipe for cakes with added fruit (see under puddings and sweet treats) for both the birthday cake and small cakes or muffins.

Fruit can be made into mini kebabs with two or three bite size chunks on cocktail sticks. Chocolate dipped fruit (see puddings and sweet treats) can be served in little sweet cases and arranged attractively on a large plate.

Drinks Serve real lemonade, high juice squash or a mixture of fruit juice and sparkling mineral water in place of the usual party soft drinks. For very special occasions you could even make junior cocktails (no alcohol, of course) using any combination of soft drinks and juices served in tall glasses with crushed ice.

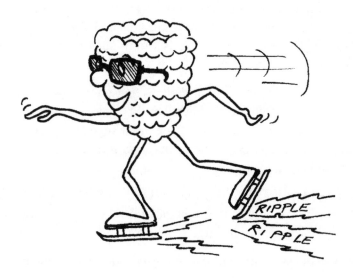

13

Eating out

Restaurant, pub and café meals for children tend to be high in fat and calories but low in nutritional content, particularly the typical kids' menu. The quality and variety of adult meals has improved considerably over the last 20 years but children's food has yet to catch up. Many national chains are recognising that parents are no longer happy with the usual chicken nuggets or burgers and some are working with nutritionists to devise healthier meals for children. Meantime, here are a few ideas to keep your child's diet as healthy as you can.

- When you plan to eat out, try to check out the menus in advance to see what they have to offer youngsters and also if they serve child sized portions of adult meals – this is one way to bypass the children's menu completely.

- Suggest to your children that perhaps they are too grown-up for the children's menu and offer them the same as mum or dad. Children do like to copy and if you order vegetables and jacket potato rather than chips and beans suggest that they might like to try this too.

- Instead of ice cream or chocolate cake for pudding, try tempting them with something that includes fruit – you can share with them if the portions are large.

- Instead of soft drinks order fruit juice or squash with the meal.

If you arrive at a pub or restaurant and the children's menu is dire, hide it while they play and order something from the adult menu that you think they will like. Alternatively, order several tempting dishes along with the right number of plates and put in the middle of the table. Tell them this is for you all to share – they can then select what they want and, with some encouragement from you, may also try new things.

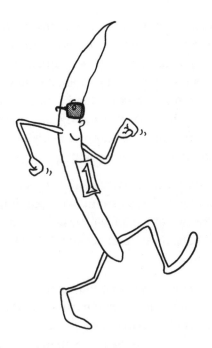

14

Holidays

Holiday food often consists of fish and chips, sandwiches and ice cream. It can be a great time but can also be stressful, particularly if children are hyperactive due to too much sugar and moody because their diet and routine have been disrupted. Constipation is often a problem too as holiday food may have little fibre. You will probably want a break from being vigilant about their diet and welcome a more relaxed time with your children. Forward planning can help things run smoothly with little effort.

- First of all, be sure to take lots of healthy snacks with you or buy a variety when you arrive for eating throughout the day. Bags of dried fruit, a variety of fresh fruit, salad for snacking and sandwiches, cereal bars, pure fruit bars and flapjacks will all provide nutrition and fibre.

- Try to start each day of your holiday with a healthy breakfast – see ideas above – so that children begin each day well. If you are staying in hotels rather than self-catering this can be more difficult and it may not be possible for them to have any fruit or vegetable portions at breakfast, so offer fruit later to supplement.

- Holidays are a great time for picnics (see packed lunches for healthier picnic ideas).

- Cakes with hidden fruit can be made in advance if you are not travelling far and removed from the freezer the day you start your holiday.

- When you have chips, whether eating out or takeaway, try to limit to two or three times a week and give children fish and pea fritters with ketchup rather than sausages and pies.

- Order fruit juice for children when you are eating out and take or buy a good supply of small fruit juice cartons for drinks throughout the day. For holiday picnics make high juice squash with some added fruit juice and real lemonade for a treat (see drinks).

- Take with you a bottle of children's vitamins and a natural laxative like syrup of figs that contains just concentrated fruit fibre. This way you can ensure that if food options are limited, children become fussy or if they lose their appetite they will have some basic nutrition and fibre.

- If you're travelling abroad you need to check whether the water, and even salads and raw foods, are safe to eat. If so, your child may be happier to experiment on holiday than at home. If they are unlikely to do so, however, take supplies of familiar foods to be sure your child doesn't go hungry.

The most important things of all, of course, are for the children to have fun and for you to relax, enjoy yourself and have a rest from the daily grind as much as is possible for parents on holiday.

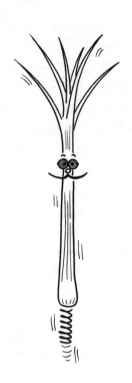

Appendix

Levels of salt recommended for children

The daily recommended maximum for children depends on their age:

- 1-3 years   2 grams salt a day (0.8g sodium)
- 4-6 years   3 grams salt a day (1.2g sodium)
- 7-10 years   5 grams salt a day (2g sodium)
- 11 and over   6 grams salt a day (2.5g sodium)

Six grams is about one teaspoon. Remember that much food consumed by children already has salt in, including baked beans, crisps and many breakfast cereals. The measurements above are the recommended maximums for children. It is better for them to have less.

Levels of sugar recommended for children

Many foods have hidden sugars, some are more obvious: an average small fruit yogurt contains four teaspoons, a can of sweetcorn contains around three quarters of a teaspoon and a can of cola contains 10 teaspoons. One bottle of fizzy drink can contain up to 15 teaspoons of sugar, more than the daily limit for a 15 year old child and twice the recommended level for a child aged 4-6. The maximum levels are slightly different for boys and girls:

- 1-3 years   29 grams (girls) 31 grams (boys)
- 4-6 years   39 grams (girls) 43 grams (boys)
- 7-10 years   43 grams (girls) 49 grams (boys)
- 11-14   46 grams (girls) 55 grams (boys)
- 15 and over   53 grams (girls) 69 grams (boys)

Further reading

An A-Z of Children's Health – A Nutritional Approach by Sally K Child, 2002, Argyll publishing, isbn 1902831403

Boost Your Child's Immune System by Lucy Burney, 2003, Piatkus, isbn 074992442X

What Really Works for Kids by Susan Clark, 2002, Bantam Press isbn 0593059195

Useful contacts

We've compiled a list of contacts, suppliers and websites which you might find useful, whether you want to find a nutritional therapist, locate some of the products recommended in this book, or find more recipes and ideas.

You'll find the list on our website at **www.whiteladderpress.com**, next to the information about this book. Keeping it online means we can keep it updated, so please let us know if we need to make any changes, or if you would like to recommend any organisation or supplier to add to the list.

If you don't have access to the internet and would like a copy of the list, call us on 01803 813343 and we'll print off a copy and send if to you.

Contact us

You're welcome to contact White Ladder Press if you have any questions or comments for either us or the authors. Please use whichever of the following routes suits you.

Phone: 01803 813343

Email: enquiries@whiteladderpress.com

Fax: 01803 813928

Address: White Ladder Press, Great Ambrook, Near Ipplepen, Devon TQ12 5UL

Website: www.whiteladderpress.com

What can our website do for you?

If you want more information about any of our books, you'll find it at www.whiteladderpress.com. In particular you'll find extracts from each of our books, and reviews of those that are already published. We also run special offers on future titles if you order online before publication. And you can request a copy of our free catalogue.

Many of our books also have links pages, useful addresses and so on relevant to the subject of the book. You'll also find out a bit more about us and, if you're a writer yourself, you'll find our submission guidelines for authors. So please check us out and let us know if you have any comments, questions or suggestions.

Fancy another good read?

If you've enjoyed this book, how about reading another of our books for helping busy parents have an easier and more enjoyable time with their children? *Kids & Co* by Ros Jay is for parents with children anywhere between two and 18, who don't always do what you want them to.

If that sounds familiar, you'll find *Kids & Co* full of useful tips and advice on using business skills (yes, really) to help you manage, motivate and negotiate with your children. You'll discover how treating your children like customers and colleagues reduces conflict and builds mutual respect, and how teamwork skills can help your children to get on better with each other.

Over the page is a taster of what you'll find in *Kids & Co*. If you like the look of it and want to order a copy you can call us on 01803 813343 or order online at **www.whiteladderpress.com**.

"Ros Jay has had a brilliant idea, and what is more she has executed it brilliantly. *Kids & Co* is the essential handbook for any manager about to commit the act of parenthood, and a thoroughly entertaining read for everyone else." John Cleese

Kids & Co
from Negotiating Skills

Aim high

The technique: A successful negotiation depends on having room for manoeuvre. If neither of you is prepared to budge from your starting position, you haven't got the basis for a negotiation at all. And your room for manoeuvre is the space between what you start off asking for, and the bottom line you'd be prepared to settle for. So the higher you aim initially, the more scope for negotiating you have... and the better chance that you will never have to drop as low as your bottom line. So if you can afford an absolute maximum discount of 20 percent, don't start by offering 18 percent. Start with 10 percent and give yourself plenty of negotiating ground.

Your son's fifth birthday is coming up, and he wants to invite all his school friends to a big party. Your personal preference is for taking him out for a treat on his own. Or, failing that, getting someone else to host the party so you can leave the country for a few hours. You're going to have to negotiate how many people he can invite.

You'll have to think about this one first, and decide what your bottom line is. Perhaps you feel you can just about cope with eight of the brats running around for the afternoon. But you can't start by offering him eight, or you have no room to give any ground – and that's not a negotiation. Besides, just because you can stand eight, doesn't mean you wouldn't be happier with six.

So aim high. If you can, find out how many he wants to invite (he may be unpractised enough in negotiating to reveal this information). You often tend to meet in the middle on this kind of deal, so if you know how many he wants, you can try to make sure eight is the middle point. If he has a list of 10, you can stipulate a maximum of six. Then you can meet in the middle at eight. If his list has 12 names on it and you start out saying six, you can't arrive at eight unless he gives more ground than you do. And how easy will that be to negotiate? So if he wants 12, you can start at four. And if you give other concessions too (as we'll see later), you might end up with even fewer than eight.

Yes, I realise that if he wants to invite 20 friends this system isn't going to be foolproof. But the odds are that he knows perfectly well 20 is unrealistic. And, as we'll see, there are other variables you can bring into play. If you have no idea how many people he wants to invite, and you can't wheedle a figure out of him – simply aim high. Suggest he invites his two or three closest friends and be prepared to give a fair bit of ground if you have to.

Remember that you need to start by aiming high, because once you've agreed to lower your demands, you can't raise them again. Imagine saying to an employee in the middle of negotiating their pay rise, "Sorry, but actually I can't offer you that five percent pay rise I said I could after all. Three percent is my absolute limit." It's just not on. You can't promise your son seven friends at his party and then reduce it to four later. Your life wouldn't be worth living.

So the one remaining question is: how high should you aim? And the answer is simple. As high as you can justify. If you ask your boss to draft in five extra staff to help you cover the exhibition next month, you know you have to be able to justify why you need five rather than only three or four. Well, the same goes here. How few friends can you justify allowing your son to invite? Think about other parties he's been to, or what he wants this party to entail, and decide what you can get away with.

It's the same with your nine year old's bedtime. You'll have a hard time justifying a bedtime of 6.30, but consider when their older siblings go to bed, what time they have to get up in the mornings, what time they go to bed now, and come up with the earliest bed-time you can reasonably justify. You're being kind really – you're giving them the chance to beat you down even further.

Look for variables

The technique: If you have only one factor to consider, such as money, you're not really negotiating at all. You're haggling. You offer 10 thousand, they say they'll take 12, you suggest 11 thousand and it's a deal. But a negotiation is more subtle and complex because you can bring in other factors, or variables. Suppose they say they'll take 12 thousand, and you say you'll give them 11 if they can deliver within three weeks. Now you're juggling cost and deliv-ery time, and you're into a true negotiation. The more of these variables you can find, the more bargaining levers you have.

It's always worth bringing in as many variables as you can to a negotiation, especially if you haven't much room for manoeuvre on the central point at issue. If bedtime is currently 9 o'clock and you're really not prepared to move far on it at all, it will help if you can introduce other factors. Maybe you can offer a later bedtime at weekends and in the holidays, or perhaps you could let them leave the light on until 10 o'clock. Or let them have one later night each week if there's a particular television programme they want to watch. You could even offer to throw in a new set of more grown-up bedding (covered in footballers rather than elephants).

You can be as creative as you like. So long as you can make offers which will appeal to your child, any variable factor like this can help to clinch a deal. If you have both reached your bottom line and still haven't met in the middle, variables can be the only way to find a workable solution. The thing is, the variables can influ-ence the bottom line. You're still set on a 9.30 bedtime, but it does-n't have to apply at weekends. They still want to go to bed at 10, but might concede four out of five weekdays.

One of the advantages of variables, however, is that they often help you to avoid ever reaching your bottom line. With no other bargaining points in play, you might have to let your five year old push you to letting him invite eight friends to his party. But introduce variables to the negotiation, and you may well keep him to fewer. For example:

- For every person he knocks off his invitation list, you'll add £20 to the budget for the party (if you're going to use bribery, you might as well be creative with it)

- If there are no more than two friends (let him negotiate you up to three here) you'll take them all out for a special treat such as the circus or a pantomime

- The fewer party guests, the longer the party can go on (put it this way to be positive, rather than saying the more there are, the shorter it will have to be)

- He can have eight people on the condition that none of them is either Jim or Matt, each of whom count as two people (and that's being generous)

Anything which will help you to reach an agreement is OK. It doesn't have to have anything to do with the matter under negotiation, so long as you are both prepared to bargain with it. So you might say that if he limits the number of friends he invites, you'll have his bike resprayed the colour he keeps asking you to.

You can be endlessly creative with variables once you get into practice. Here's another standard negotiation which all of us have to hold with our children sooner or later: pocket money. Instead of simply haggling, think of some more variables:

- Half their pocket money is sacrosanct, the other half has to be earned by doing chores

- They can't have the raise they want, but you'll give them a book allowance every month as well

- Pocket money can go up, but they have to save a percentage of it towards more expensive items which you approve (they can always save the rest of it towards things you don't approve)

...and so on. I'm sure you've got the idea.

Just don't limit yourself. You have far more scope when it comes to negotiating with your children than with your customers or your boss, because you should have a much better idea of what will motivate them, even if it's unrelated to the subject under discussion. After all, you can't generally sway a customer by saying "Oh, and if you'll settle for a 15 percent discount, I'll take you camping on Saturday night."

Recipes *for* Disaster*s*

How to turn kitchen cock-ups into magnificent meals

Roni Jay

"Methinks 'twould have spared me much grief had I had this cunning volume to hand when I burnt those cursèd cakes." *King Alfred the Great*

It was all going so well... friends for lunch, guests for dinner, family for Christmas. You're planning a delicious meal, relaxed yet sophisticated, over which everyone can chat, drink a glass of fine wine and congratulate you on your culinary talent.

And then, just as you were starting to enjoy it – disaster! The pastry has burnt, the pudding has collapsed or the terrine won't turn out. Or the main ingredient has been eaten by the cat. Or perhaps it's the guests who've buggered everything up: they forgot to mention that they're vegetarian (you've made a beef bourguignon). Or they've brought along a friend (you've only made six crème brûlées).

But don't panic. There are few kitchen cock-ups that can't be successfully salvaged if you know how. With the right attitude you are no longer accident-prone, but adaptable. Not a panicker but a creative, inspirational cook. Recipes for Disasters is packed with useful tips and ideas for making sure that your entertaining always runs smoothly (or at least appears to, whatever is going on behind the scenes). Yes, you still can have a reputation as a culinary paragon, even if it is all bluff.

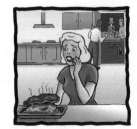

£7.99

HOW TO SURVIVE THE TERRIBLE TWOS

Diary of a mother under siege

CAROLINE DUNFORD

Living with a two-year-old isn't necessarily easy. In fact, your child's second year is as steep a learning curve for you as it is for them. While they're finding out about the world, you're struggling to get to grips with everything from food fads to potty training, sleepless nights to choosing a playgroup.

Caroline Dunford has charted a year in the life of her two-year-old son, aptly known as the Emperor on account of his transparent master plan to bend the known universe to his will. She recounts her failures as honestly as her successes, and passes on what she's learnt about:

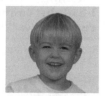

- how to get a decent night's sleep
- coaxing a half decent diet down your toddler
- keeping your child safe, at home and beyond
- getting your child out of nappies
- curing bad habits, from spitting and hitting to hair pulling and head-banging

...and plenty more of the everyday sagas and traumas that beset any parent of a two-year-old. This real life account reassures you that you're not alone, and gives you plenty of suggestions and guidance to make this year feel more like peaceful negotiation than a siege.

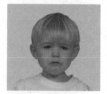

Caroline Dunford has previously worked as a psychotherapist, a counsellor, a supervisor, a writer and a tutor – sometimes concurrently. Even working three jobs at once did not, in any way, prepare her for the onset of motherhood. Today she is a mother and, when her son allows, a freelance writer.

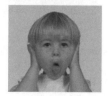

£7.99

What every parent should know *before* their child goes to university

Jane Bidder

Starting at uni is daunting, worrying, stressful. Not for them, for you. They want to appear independent, but secretly they still want support. So where does that leave you?

What Every Parent Should Know Before Their Child Goes to University charts your route through the new parental territory you're about to enter. It draws on the experience of parents who have gone before you to help with:

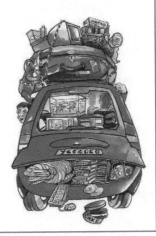

- how to fill in those UCAS forms
- changing courses, or even changing uni
- organising accommodation
- what to pack, and other essentials
- money and teaching them to budget
- coping with the changes for you at home
- problems from stress to sex, homesickness to drugs, term time jobs to broken hearts

£9.99

Order form

You can order any of our books via any of the contact routes on page 106, including on our website. Or fill out the order form below and fax it or post it to us.

We'll normally send your copy out by first class post within 24 hours (but please allow five days for delivery). We don't charge postage and packing within the UK. Please add £1 per book for postage outside the UK.

Title (Mr/Mrs/Miss/Ms/Dr/Lord etc) _____

Name _____

Address _____

Postcode _____

Daytime phone number _____

Email _____

No. of copies	Title	Price	Total £
	Postage and packing £1 per book (outside the UK only):		
	TOTAL:		

Please either send us a cheque made out to White Ladder Press Ltd or fill in the credit card details below.

Type of card ☐ Visa ☐ Mastercard ☐ Switch

Card number _____

Start date (if on card) _____ Expiry date _____ Issue no (Switch) _____

Name as shown on card _____

Signature _____

Index of Recipes